THE ENVIRONMENTAL IMPACT OF MERCURY-CONTAINING DENTAL AMALGAMS

HEARING

BEFORE THE

SUBCOMMITTEE ON HUMAN RIGHTS AND WELLNESS

OF THE

COMMITTEE ON GOVERNMENT REFORM

HOUSE OF REPRESENTATIVES

ONE HUNDRED EIGHTH CONGRESS

FIRST SESSION

OCTOBER 8, 2003

Serial No. 108–102

Printed for the use of the Committee on Government Reform

Available via the World Wide Web: http://www.gpo.gov/congress/house
http://www.house.gov/reform

U.S. GOVERNMENT PRINTING OFFICE

91–841 PDF   WASHINGTON : 2004

CONTENTS

THE ENVIRONMENTAL IMPACT OF MERCURY-CONTAINING DENTAL AMALGAMS

WEDNESDAY, OCTOBER 8, 2003

House of Representatives,
Subcommittee on Human Rights and Wellness,
Committee on Government Reform,
Washington, DC.

The subcommittee met, pursuant to notice, at 4 p.m., in room 2157, Rayburn House Office Building, Hon. Dan Burton (chairman of the subcommittee) presiding.

Present: Representatives Burton and Cummings.

Staff present: Mark Walker, staff director; John Rowe and Brian Fauls, professional staff member; Danielle Perraut, clerk; Nick Mutton, press secretary; Richard Butcher, minority professional staff member; and Cecelia Morton, minority office manager.

Mr. Burton. A quorum being present, the Subcommittee on Human Rights and Wellness will come to order. I ask unanimous consent that all Members and witnesses' written and opening statements be included in the record. Without objection, so ordered. I ask unanimous consent that all articles, exhibits and extraneous or tabular material referred to be included in the record. Without objection, so ordered.

Recently, there was an incident at a local high school here in D.C. that rightfully received front page news and that dramatically illustrates the danger of mercury toxicity. Just last week, several students walked into an unlocked chemistry lab, stole a vial of mercury and decided to splash it all over the floors and walls of the school. The result was an immediate evacuation and closure of the building. The building could be closed for as long as 4 months while authorities work to ensure that all traces of the mercury have been eliminated. During the extensive cleanup process, students will have to attend classes in uncontaminated buildings and they have been instructed to turn in the clothes that they were wearing and their shoes that they wore that day of the incident to have them decontaminated.

[The information referred to follows:]

The Washington Post

washingtonpost.com

The Washington Post

October 07, 2003, Tuesday, Final Edition

SECTION: METRO; Pg. B05

LENGTH: 1054 words

HEADLINE: Students at Ballou Bused Elsewhere After Screenings; Cleanup Continues After **Mercury Spill**

BYLINE: Manny Fernandez and David A. Fahrenthold, Washington Post Staff Writers

BODY:
Ballou Senior High School in Southeast Washington resumed classes yesterday after last week's **mercury spill,** but the school day was anything but normal.

Hundreds of students spent most of the morning waiting in a block-long line for mercury contamination screening in the parking lot in an area set up by federal and local authorities. Parents who had taken time off from work talked in clusters, and administrators scrambled to bus pupils to temporary classrooms at a nearby school and at the old Washington Convention Center downtown.

"We'll get through it," Ballou Principal Art Bridges said as he patrolled the line of youths along the school's chain-link fence on Fourth Street SE, bullhorn in hand. "My students are bold, courageous and outstanding. They will achieve."

Ballou was evacuated and then shuttered Thursday after the potentially poisonous metal was stolen from an unlocked science laboratory and spread throughout the school, in the gym, cafeteria, hallways and several classrooms. More than 20 Ballou students may have handled some of the liquid, D.C. police said. Cmdr. Winston Robinson, who heads the 7th Police District, said various groups of students had carried the material, a silvery substance that Robinson said reminded some students of a special effect in the Arnold Schwarzenegger action movie "Terminator 2: Judgment Day."

"The kids didn't realize what the liquid was, and they were actually holding the liquid, rolling it around," Robinson said. One student told police he carried the mercury on a napkin, while other students carried it on pieces of paper. At one point, Robinson said, the chemical was taken outside the school, where students were throwing it at one another. Officials said they did not know how much mercury had been stored in the unused honors chemistry lab, which was scheduled for renovation, but said at least 250 milliliters, or about a cupful, was taken.

Officers have identified one student who they say was involved in taking the mercury from the lab, and Robinson said the student was interviewed by detectives. For now, he said, police are not treating the incident as a criminal matter. William Wilhoyte, assistant superintendent for high schools, said that the students involved did not intend to disrupt school and that the incident was a case of "kids being kids." Bridges reiterated yesterday that the student or students involved would not be suspended but would receive "a stern talking-to" or some type of in-school punishment.

Yesterday's three-hour screening and ongoing building cleanup represented an unprecedented disruption for the students, parents, faculty and staff of the 1,300-student school. A multi-agency team, including the federal Environmental Protection Agency, the city health department, the D.C. public schools and others, is working to clean up the building, to screen students and employees and to investigate the spill.

Marcos Aquino, on-scene coordinator for the EPA, said the cleanup could take weeks. So school officials have turned the old convention center site into a makeshift schoolhouse, setting up 33 classrooms inside meeting rooms and opening a nurse's station and teacher's lounge in the barren but still carpeted facility. They also trucked in photocopying machines, tables, chairs, textbooks and other materials.

EPA officials said their time estimates were based on other mercury cleanups they have conducted in the mid-Atlantic region over the past several years. "We'd rather take our time to ensure that the cleanup is properly done and complete, rather than worry about a time frame and let the kids in before it's deemed safe," said Patricia L. Taylor, EPA community involvement coordinator.

The screening process began yesterday about 8:15 a.m., with faculty and staff going first and students following, Aquino said. Students were told to place clothes and shoes they had worn Thursday in a sealed plastic bag and take the bag to school. Those being screened sat on metal folding chairs in one of four stations in the parking lot, and a suitcase-like machine with a hose attached was used to check for mercury vapor on their clothes and shoes. They then talked briefly with city health officials as part of an epidemiological study. The students were put on Metro and charter buses and driven to class. Ninth-graders were taken to nearby Charles Hart Middle School, and the rest of the student body was bused to the convention center.

About 730 faculty members, students and staff members were screened for mercury vapors yesterday as the cleanup continued inside the building. About 250 plastic bags of clothing and shoes were collected for analysis.

Michael S.A. Richardson, the District's chief medical officer, said that 80 bags of belongings were retained for further testing, and that 10 students and two adults exhibited symptoms of an ailment. Only five of those with symptoms showed signs suggesting mercury exposure, he said. A serious, large exposure to liquid mercury can damage the lungs, kidneys and central nervous system, but officials said there was no evidence last night that any such exposure had occurred at Ballou.

D.C. school officials said they were pleased that the screening process and the few hours of instruction they were able to provide students had gone smoothly.

The screening will take place again today so officials can make sure that all students and staff who were at the school Thursday go through the examination process. School officials said about 900 of the 1,300 students were in attendance Thursday. Students are to report at 8:45 a.m. at Ballou, where they will be escorted to Hart or driven to the convention center.

Some parents expressed frustration that the screening was not done sooner and wanted answers as to why the room where the chemicals were stored was unlocked. "That classroom should have been locked down," said the mother of a ninth-grader who came to Ballou to monitor the situation, as did others.

Richardson said officials are looking into whether proper procedures in the handling and storage of the chemical were followed at the school. School officials dispatched teams to all

other public high schools and middle schools to ensure that mercury and other chemicals
have been stored properly.

LOAD-DATE: October 07, 2003

Document 1 of 11 next ▶

Mr. BURTON. I am sure that everyone here today would agree that these precautions make perfect sense in order to safeguard and protect the health of the students, teachers and staff. I personally believe that there is no more important function of government than doing everything in its power to protect the health and well-being of its citizens. That is why as chairman of the House Committee on Government Reform and now the chairman of the Subcommittee on Human Rights and Wellness, I have led a 2-year-long investigation into the dangers of using highly toxic mercury in everyday medical and dental procedures.

Mercury is one of the most toxic elements found in nature, second only to radioactive materials. While some minerals are beneficial to human life, mercury is most assuredly not, because the human body was not designed or ever meant to ingest mercury. Consequently, the human body has no effective filter or elimination system for it. The end result is that much of the ingested mercury accumulates in the body's tissue, including the nervous system and vital organs, such as the brain.

Previous committee and subcommittee hearings have focused on the dangers of mercury-containing thimerosal in vaccines and mercury-containing dental amalgam fillings. In each case, credible witnesses provided clear and convincing scientific testimony that links mercury in the human body to a variety of developmental and neurological disorders from modest declines in intelligent quotient, to tremors, Alzheimer's disease and autism.

As the dangers of mercury have become more widely understood, government agencies on the Federal, State and local level have acted to eliminate mercury from common items like thermometers, blood pressure gauges, light switches, cosmetics and teething powder. Yet despite all the evidence to the contrary, mercury amalgam fillings continue to be routinely used in human dentistry. Collectively Americans are walking around today with 800 metric tons of mercury in their mouths and tens of millions of mercury-containing fillings continue to be put into Americans' teeth every single year. In spite of overwhelming evidence that mercury is especially dangerous to young children and women of child-bearing age, millions of mercury amalgams continue to be placed in their mouths every single year, and dentists cannot honestly say that they are not aware of the dangers of mercury.

In fact, dentists take routine precautions against this dangerous substance. Mercury-containing amalgam scraps and extracted teeth with amalgam fillings according to protocol must be stored in sealed jars under liquid until a special hazardous materials recycler picks them up for special disposal. Unfortunately, a lot of them get into the water supply.

If dentists are aware of the dangers of mercury, why is this toxic material still being used? The answer is that the dental establishment continues to hold to the scientific fiction that a material that is hazardous before it goes into your mouth and hazardous after it comes out of your mouth is somehow perfectly safe while it is in your mouth. This disconnect in logic simply does not make sense and it flies in the face of a growing body of credible scientific evidence.

The fact is that dentistry continues to dangerously expose humans to mercury, both through direct implantation of amalgams into patients' teeth and again during the disposal process by increasing the amount of mercury in our wastewater treatment plants.

The Association of Metropolitan Sewerage Agencies [AMSA], estimates that on average dentists contribute 35 to 40 percent of the influent mercury received by publicly owned sewerage treatment plants. In many municipalities, dentists are the highest, largest source of wastewater mercury.

And as an element, mercury remains always mercury.

Wastewater treatment plants cannot simply treat it. It must be completely removed from the wastewater system and stream.

If the mercury is not removed, heavy particles of mercury settle into treatment plant sludge. Eventually that sludge either gets incinerated, releasing its mercury directly into the atmosphere or it gets spread out on agricultural fields as fertilizer. Over time, bacteria help recirculate that mercury back into the environment. So mercury that ultimately escapes into the environment inevitably ends up in the food we eat and the air we breathe.

AMSA has estimated that it costs as much as $21 million per pound to safely remove mercury once it becomes part of the wastewater stream. If the American Dental Association's estimate is correct that approximately 6½ tons of mercury enter public wastewater treatment facilities from dental offices every year at $21 million per pound, the cost to remove that amount of mercury would be approximately $273 billion annually. That is a staggering amount of money.

A more cost effective solution in my opinion would be to simply stop the mercury contamination at its source within the dentists' offices. The technology to do just that exists today. The only thing standing in the way of using it is professional inertia.

Today's hearing will examine the facts surrounding dental amalgam's impact on the environment, discuss some cost effective measures to mitigate that impact and to promote improved mercury-safe communities for all Americans. I look forward to hearing what our expert witnesses have to say today.

Many of my colleagues because of the lateness of the hour had to catch planes, and so I apologize for them not being here. We have some of their statements which we will include in the record. I am told that Mr. Sanders and Mr. Cummings will be here shortly.

In the meantime, I would like to bring our first witnesses to the table and have them sworn. Mr. Geoffrey Grubbs, Director of the Office of Science and Technology at the EPA, and Captain James Ragain Jr. with the Dental Corps of the U.S. Navy.

Would you please stand and raise your right hands? We have two other people with you. Would you identify them?

Captain RAGAIN. Yes, sir. On my immediate left is Commander John Kuehne, U.S. Navy, and Dr. Mark Stone.

Mr. BURTON. Very good. They might participate, so I will have them raise their right hands, too.

[Witnesses sworn.]

Mr. BURTON. Mr. Grubbs, would you want to start or Captain Ragain?

STATEMENTS OF GEOFFREY GRUBBS, DIRECTOR, OFFICE OF SCIENCE AND TECHNOLOGY; AND CAPT. JAMES RAGAIN, JR., DENTAL CORPS, U.S. NAVY, ACCOMPANIED BY CDR. JOHN KUEHNE, U.S. NAVY; AND DR. MARK STONE, PROGRAM MANAGER FOR THE NIDBR MERCURY ABATEMENT PROGRAM

Mr. GRUBBS. I will be glad to start. With your permission, I would like to submit the entire statement for the record and just touch on a few quick highlights in the interest of time here.

Mercury persists in the environment and under certain conditions inorganic mercury in fresh and salt water is transformed by microorganisms into organic methylmercury. This transformation enables mercury to accumulate in the tissue of fish and other organisms. Relatively higher concentrations can be found in the top of the food chain in larger ocean going predatory fish.

Moving to the next page of my testimony so you can follow along in my skipping here, concentrations in water of mercury from all sources are low and of little immediate health concern, referring to acute toxicity problems. The greatest mercury exposure and the greatest potential risk exists for those persons who regularly eat fish containing elevated levels of methylmercury over long periods of time. Approximately 8 percent of reproductive aged women in a recent study conducted by the Centers for Disease Control within HHS had blood mercury concentrations higher than a safe level based on EPA's reference dose and that is the level that EPA has determined is safe. Forty-four States, one territory and three tribes have issued fish consumption advisories for mercury contaminated fish, all of whom are based, or nearly all of them are based on EPA's advice.

I am going to skip to the section marked Mercury in Dental Waste on page 3. Dental amalgam contributes a small proportion of all mercury released to the environment from human activities. Virtually all releases of dental amalgam to water are through municipal wastewater facilities. A recent study by the American Metropolitan Sewerage Authorities found that dental clinics account for an average of more than 35 percent of the mercury influent to the sewerage treatment plants.

An American Dental Association survey indicates that in 1996 the dental industry used 31 metric tons of mercury. The majority of waste dental mercury amalgam from chairside drains is removed by traps and vacuum filters but according to several reports, 25 to 40 percent of the mercury-containing amalgam waste is discharged to sewer systems. The physical processes used in sewerage treatment plants remove about 95 percent of the mercury received in wastewater. The mercury removed from wastewater then resides in the biosolids or it is sometimes called sludges generated during primary and secondary treatment processes. EPA estimates that sewage sludge nationally contains about 15 tons of mercury per year and this is from all sources, not just from dental amalgam. Sewerage treatment plants discharge about a half a ton of mercury to surface waters per year nationally, again from all sources.

We do not know exactly the proportion of mercury that is found in fish originates in dental amalgam as compared to other mercury sources. The mercury contained in amalgam is not methylmercury and tends to stay bound in the amalgam. However, dental amalgam can break down and at least one report has shown that it can be released into the environment.

The amount of mercury from dental amalgams that is methylated is not currently known. The American Dental Association has identified numerous best management practices for reducing mercury waste from dental amalgam, including chairside screens and traps. Amalgam separators are available at a relatively low cost to remove fine particles of waste amalgam. The choice of dental treatment rests solely with dental professionals and their patients and EPA does not intend to second-guess those treatment decisions. However, over time as fewer mercury-containing dental amalgams are used in favor of composites, amalgam will become less of a source of mercury in the environment.

Turning to EPA actions, EPA is working on a mercury action plan to describe EPA's long-term goals and near-term priority actions involving mercury in all media and under all of EPA's statutory authorities. Under the Clean Air Act in the United States, we have cut emissions by over 90 percent from two of the largest categories of sources of airborne mercury, municipal waste combustion and medical waste incineration. These are through maximum achievable control technology requirements.

The United States also has a goal under the Great Lakes Binational Strategy which we executed with the country of Canada to reduce mercury emissions and water releases by 50 percent from 1990 levels. That would be done by 2006.

The administration has proposed the clear skies legislation that would create a mandatory program to reduce from power plants emissions of mercury, sulfur dioxide and nitrogen oxides, and in this proposal mercury emissions would be cut by 70 percent by the year 2018.

Under the Clean Water Act, which is primarily where I work, through the NPDES discharge permit program, those are regulatory permits issued to all dischargers and the national pretreatment programs which sewerage treatment plants need to deal with. EPA and authorized States encourage sewerage treatment plants to develop and implement pollution prevention strategies to reduce the amount of mercury received by the wastewater treatment plant. There are several examples of that we can provide to you.

The Clean Water Act requires EPA to develop scientific information on safe levels of pollution and for States to adopt water quality standards for open and ambient water that protect human health and the environment. In January 2001, EPA published a new ambient water quality criterion recommendation for methylmercury which is expressed as a fish and shellfish tissue value rather than as an ambient water column value. States are now starting to adopt this new water quality criterion into their water quality standards.

EPA has also promulgated water quality standards for the Great Lakes and their tributaries which take into account the effects of mercury on birds and mammals that consume contaminated fish. The Clean Water Act also requires States to assess their waters periodically to determine whether those water bodies exceed ambient water quality standards and, if they do exceed them, to establish total maximum daily loads for those waters. Total maximum daily loads are basically a budget which lays out who needs to do what, including regulatory requirements, in order to meet the ambient goal of the water quality standard.

States have so far identified 1,097 water bodies where the levels of mercury exceed their water quality standards, and so far States have completed 144 TMDLs for these water bodies. EPA also has a research program that is primarily invested in the fate and transport as well as other areas to address science needs for mercury. We are funding that at the level of $5.5 million per year.

With that, I will end my statement. I would be glad to expand on any of these quick highlights as we turn to questions and to answer any questions you might have.

[The prepared statement of Mr. Grubbs follows:]

STATEMENT OF
GEOFFREY GRUBBS
DIRECTOR, OFFICE OF SCIENCE AND TECHNOLOGY
U.S. ENVIRONMENTAL PROTECTION AGENCY
BEFORE THE
SUBCOMMITTEE ON WELLNESS AND HUMAN RIGHTS
OF THE
COMMITTEE ON GOVERNMENT REFORM
UNITED STATES HOUSE OF REPRESENTATIVES

October 8, 2003

Good afternoon, Mr. Chairman and Members of the Subcommittee. I am Geoffrey

Grubbs, Director of the Office of Science and Technology in the Office of Water, at the U.S.

Environmental Protection Agency (EPA). I appreciate this opportunity to discuss mercury in

dental amalgam and how we believe it may affect our nation's waters.

INTRODUCTION

Mercury is an element which occurs in the natural environment. Mercury persists in the

environment and, under certain conditions, inorganic mercury in fresh and salt water is

transformed by microorganisms into organic methylmercury. This transformation enables mercury

to accumulate in the tissue of fish and other organisms that are part of the food web. While

methylmercury can be found in virtually all fish and many marine mammals, relatively higher

concentrations can be found at the top of the food chain in larger ocean going predatory fish.

Dental amalgam contributes a small proportion of all mercury released to the environment

from human activities. Virtually all releases of dental amalgam are through municipal waste water

facilities, and EPA estimates that sewage sludge nationally contains about 15 tons of mercury per

year. A recent study by the American Metropolitan Sewerage Authorities (AMSA) found that

dental clinics account for an average of more than 35 percent of the mercury influent to the seven

POTWs studied, more than four times the percentage contributed by the next largest source categories - human waste and hospitals.

Concentrations of mercury in water are low and of little immediate health concern. The greatest mercury exposure and potential risk exists for those persons who regularly eat fish containing elevated levels of methylmercury over long periods of time. The Centers for Disease Control (CDC) and Prevention's National Report on Human Exposure to Environmental Chemicals support the conclusion from an NRC committee review based on earlier estimates of methylmercury exposure in U.S. populations that *in utero* methylmercury exposure is low. However, approximately 8% of reproductive-aged women in the CDC study have blood mercury concentrations higher than a safe level based on EPA's reference dose (that is the level EPA considers to be safe). These elevated levels may constitute a risk to a developing child in the womb, although none of these women had blood mercury concentrations at the substantially higher levels known to present such a risk. Forty-four states, one territory and three tribes have issued fish consumption advisories for mercury-contaminated fish. Fish advisory information is not a surrogate for exposure to the general population because many people eat only commercial fish that they purchase in stores or restaurants. However, there are subpopulations who do consume fish they have caught from waters covered by fish advisories. EPA and the Food and Drug Administration are working together to develop a joint fish consumption advisory on the risks to women of childbearing age and young children from methylmercury in commercial and locally caught fish.

The Clean Air Act and the Clean Water Act (CWA) authorize EPA to limit releases of mercury to air and water. For example, the CWA requires the National Pollutant Discharge

Elimination System (NPDES) permits that specify effluent limitations where necessary to protect water quality. For municipal waste water treatment plants (i.e., Publicly Owned Treatment Works [POTWs]) that are subject to these effluent limitations, the National Pretreatment Program requires control of commercial and industrial sources of pollutants in influents.

MERCURY IN DENTAL WASTE

Dental amalgam contributes a small proportion of all mercury released to the environment from human activities. Virtually all releases of dental amalgam are through municipal waste water facilities. A recent study by the American Metropolitan Sewerage Authorities (AMSA) found that dental clinics account for an average of more than 35 percent of the mercury influent to the seven POTWs studied, more than four times the percentage contributed by the next largest source categories - human waste and hospitals. This study did not estimate the total national amount of mercury entering POTWs, only the relative loading for the POTWs studied. An American Dental Association survey indicates that in 1996, the dental industry used 31 metric tons of mercury. Amalgam for dental fillings contains about 50% mercury, with silver and other metals constituting the remaining portion.

Mercury-containing amalgam wastes may find their way to the environment in two ways. When new fillings are placed, waste amalgam material enters the solid waste stream, and waste particles from the placement process may be flushed into chairside drains. When old mercury-containing fillings are drilled out, fine particles of amalgam also may be flushed into chairside drains. The majority of the waste dental amalgam from chairside drains is removed by traps and vacuum filters. But, according to reports, 25 to 40 percent (Riversides Stewardship Alliance, 2001, "Campaigns: Mercury Free Dentists", and Cailas, M.D., Ovsey, V.G., Mihailova, C.,

Naleway, C., Batch, H., Fan, P.L., Chou, H-N, Stone, M., Mayer, D., Ralls, S., Roddy, W.:

"Physico-chemical Properties of Dental Wastewater"; Water Environment Federation 67th Annual

Conference & Exposition, Chicago, IL, 1994) of the mercury-containing amalgam waste is

discharged to sewer systems. Some of the waste amalgam particles that reach the sewer system

settle out in the sewers and some are carried to POTWs.

The physical processes used in POTWs remove about 95% of the mercury received in

waste water. The mercury removed from waste water then resides in the biosolids or sludges

generated during primary and secondary treatment processes. EPA estimates that sewage sludge

nationally contains about 15 tons of mercury per year. This is based on levels of mercury

reported by EPA in the National Sewage Sludge Survey (55 F.R. 47210-47283, 1990) and EPA

reports of POTW sludge use and disposal practices (Proposed Part 503 Standards for the

Disposal of Sewage Sludge, EPA, Feb. 6, 1989). POTWs discharge about a half ton of mercury

to surface waters per year nationally. Some of the mercury in sludge can return to the

environment through sludge incineration.

We do not know exactly the proportion of mercury found in fish which originates from

dental amalgam as compared to other mercury sources. The mercury contained in amalgam is not

methylmercury and tends to stay bound in the amalgam under most environmental conditions

(Arenholt-Bindslev and Larsen, "Mercury Levels and Discharge in Waste Water from Dental

Clinics," Water, Air, and Soil Pollution, Vol. 86, pp. 93-99). However, dental amalgam can break

down and release mercury into the environment (MAREK, M. 1990. The Release of Mercury

from Dental Amalgam: The Mechanisms and *In Vitro* Testing. J. Dent. Res. 69: 1167-1174; other studies corroborate this finding.) The amount of mercury from dental amalgams that is methylated is not currently known.

Taking measures to prevent the dental amalgam from getting into the water in the first place, reduces the amount of dental amalgam and thus decreases mercury in waste water. The American Dental Association has identified numerous Best Management Practices for reducing mercury wastes from dental amalgam, including chairside screens and traps.   Amalgam separators are also available at relatively low cost to remove fine particles of waste amalgam. A number of studies, including one conducted by EPA's Environmental Technology Verification Program, show a high degree of effectiveness of separators. Amalgam separators and other practices in dental offices can reduce the amount of mercury discharged to POTWs.

Another way to reduce the amount of amalgam entering the sewers is for dentists to use mercury-free fillings. The cost to patients of mercury-free fillings however, have been reported to be 1.5 to 8 times more than amalgam. Insurance companies may be unwilling to pay these additional costs.

The choice of dental treatment rests solely with dental professionals and their patients. EPA does not intend to second-guess these treatment decisions. Alternatives to mercury containing dental amalgams exist. As fewer mercury-containing dental amalgams are provided as treatment, they will become less of a source of mercury in the environment.

EPA ACTIONS

EPA is committed to achieving a better understanding and reduction of the public health risk to our nation's citizens with respect to mercury. EPA is working on a Mercury Action Plan to guide the Agency to an increasingly holistic and integrated approach to reducing mercury exposure, and will include the actions discussed below. When final, this Mercury Action Plan will describe EPA's long-term goals and near-term priority actions, based on available scientific information on health and environmental impacts of mercury exposure and on the current status of EPA's program activities. In addition, the action plan's holistic perspective and approach to mercury also will be useful to other federal agencies, states, industry, academia, and the public in addressing mercury.

EPA has substantially limited emissions of mercury to the atmosphere through a Maximum Achievable Control Technology requirement under the Clean Air Act. As a result, the U.S. has cut emissions by over 90% from two of the three largest categories of sources, municipal waste combustion and medical waste incineration. Additionally, the U.S. has a goal under the Great Lakes Binational Strategy (U.S.-Canada) to reduce mercury emissions and water releases by 50% from 1990 levels and reduce use of mercury through regulatory and voluntary mercury reduction programs. EPA expects that these actions will reduce levels of mercury in air, and thus reduce the amount of mercury that eventually finds its way into rivers and lakes.

The Administration has proposed the Clear Skies legislation that would create a mandatory program to reduce power plant emissions of mercury, sulfur dioxide and nitrogen oxides by setting a national cap on each pollutant. It would cut mercury emissions by nearly 70 percent. Emissions would be cut from 1999 levels of 48 tons by a cap of 26 tons in 2010 and a cap of 15 tons in 2018.

Direct releases of mercury to water bodies are controlled through programs under the Clean Water Act, including NPDES permits issued by authorized states and EPA. AMSA estimates that six percent (253 of 4,307) of the NPDES permits issued to major POTWs include mercury effluent limits. AMSA also estimates that ten percent (423 of 4,307) of these discharge permits have monitoring requirements.

Through the NPDES permit and the National Pretreatment Programs, EPA encourages POTWs to develop and implement pollution prevention strategies to reduce the amount of mercury received by the wastewater treatment plant. Effective mercury source reduction relies on the POTW effectively communicating to sector entities the fact that small scale individual efforts can collectively reduce the mercury loading to the environment. Forming partnerships and working with sector representatives to investigate mercury sources, explore alternatives, and assist in implementation of selected options is integral to a successful reduction strategy. For example, the Western Lake Superior Sanitary District determined that one industry and many small other sources, including dental facilities, contributed a major portion of the mercury in their wastewater. With respect to dental offices, the local POTW in Duluth, Minnesota, worked with the local dental offices to produce a manual containing BMPs on proper disposal of mercury in amalgam. Monitoring by the POTW shows that the amount of mercury discharges from dental offices has been reduced by over two-thirds.

In addition, the CWA requires EPA to develop scientific information on safe levels of pollution and for States to adopt water quality standards that protect public health and the environment. In January 2001, EPA published a new ambient water quality criterion recommendation for methylmercury which is expressed as a fish and shellfish tissue value rather than as an ambient water column value. This criterion of 0.3 parts per million (ppm) represents EPA's best scientific understanding of the level of mercury in fish tissue that will not lead to adverse effects to the average eater of fish. States are starting to adopt new criteria in their water quality standards based on EPA's recommendation of 0.3 ppm to update their current standards.

As part of our overall goal to protect water, EPA issued a final rule in 1995 that puts in place water quality standards for the Great Lakes and their tributaries. This is the first time water quality standards took into account the effects of mercury on birds and mammals that consume contaminated fish, and serves to provide a more comprehensive level of protection for the environment.

In addition to NPDES permits and water quality standards, the CWA requires States to assess their waters to determine if they exceed water quality standards and if they do, to establish Total Maximum Daily Loads (TMDLs) for those waters. States have identified 1,097 (1998 and 2000 data) waterbodies where the levels of mercury exceed their water quality standards. States and EPA are developing TMDLs that identify the necessary reductions in mercury loadings to achieve these standards. To date, 144 are done. Some TMDLs are implemented through NPDES permits and others are designed so as to prevent increases in current mercury loadings to prevent impairments of waters.

EPA has a strategically targeted mercury research program focusing on priority areas, including transport and fate of mercury. EPA's Mercury Research Multi-Year Plan identifies as one of its two major long range goals the achievement of "an understanding of the transport and fate of mercury from release to receptor and its effects on the receptor." Resources for the implementation of the research activities in this plan total about $5.5 million annually to be spent on various areas, including transport and fate, using both Science to Achieve Results (STAR) funds and in-house research. Between 1999 and 2005, the STAR grants program has committed approximately $13 million for atmospheric and aquatic transport and fate research.

CONCLUSION

I commend this subcommittee for conducting a hearing on this important topic. We look forward to continuing to discuss these important issues with you.

Thank you. I look forward to your questions.

* * *

Mr. BURTON. Thank you. Before we go to Captain Ragain, do you have an opening statement you would like to make, Mr. Cummings?

Mr. CUMMINGS. I do, Mr. Chairman, but why don't we go to the next witness.

Mr. BURTON. Captain Ragain.

Captain RAGAIN. Mr. Chairman, Honorable Representatives, ladies and gentlemen, good afternoon. Thank you for inviting us to testify before the Subcommittee on Human Rights and Wellness. I am Captain James C. Ragain Jr., Dental Corps, U.S. Navy, Commanding Officer of the Naval Institute for Dental and Biomedical Research [NIDBR], located at the Naval Service Training Center, Great Lakes, IL. Accompanying me this afternoon are Commander John C. Kuehne, Dental Corps, head of the Bioenvironmental Sciences Department, and Dr. Mark E. Stone, program manager for the NIDBR Mercury Abatement Program.

NIDBR's research related to the control of mercury emissions from dental amalgam began in 1991 as a collaboration with the American Dental Association involving the evaluation of commercial amalgam separators. NIDBR instituted a mercury management program to coordinate and direct the research efforts of a number of dental researchers and equipment specialists. This program made great strides in the design and installation of pretreatment systems at several Navy dental treatment facilities. NIDBR was then designated by Navy dentistry as the lead agent for development, evaluation and guidance regarding Navy wide installation of pretreatment systems to minimize the environmental impact of Navy dentistry.

The tasking required that pretreatment systems be able to remove mercury in order to allow all Navy dental clinics to comply with local wastewater discharge standards. NIDBR was specifically tasked to assess current compliance of dental treatment facilities [DTFs], in meeting local discharge standards and to develop strategies to bring all DTFs in the Navy into compliance. This includes ships, field and mobile dental units.

In fiscal year 2001, NIDBR began the implementation of a multiyear program to survey and install pretreatment systems in every Navy DTF worldwide. To date, pretreatment systems of various sizes have been successfully installed in 50 percent of all Navy dental clinics located within the continental United States. By the end of calendar year 2003, we expect to have completed the installation of mercury abatement systems in 95 percent of the Navy's U.S. clinics. These systems meet local discharge limits with anywhere from 95 to greater than 99 percent of total mercury removed from the wastewater.

Previously completed wastewater characterization studies by NIDBR have enabled us to develop a pretreatment strategy that allows for the removal of mercury to extremely low levels, thus reducing mercury from grams per liter to micrograms per liter in the waste stream.

NIDBR's strategy involves the phased treatment of the dental-unit wastewater stream. Phase 1 is the removal of amalgam particulate through filtration and/or settling. Removal of particulate greater than 10 microns removes up to 95 percent of the total mercury in the waste stream. However, a significant amount of mercury is located in the dissolved or soluble fraction and is high enough to violate some local discharge limits. In phase 2, the remaining dissolved mercury is driven to the ionic form by oxidation and removed by sorbents. This phased treatment program has proved very effective for both large and small dental treatment facilities. An additional benefit of the phased pretreatment strategy is the ability to deploy technology that can be scaled to meet variable local water treatment facilities' discharge limits.

Navy dentistry's mercury abatement program is a proactive effort intended to keep the Navy in compliance with local and overseas environmental requirements, and the successful implementation of these pretreatment systems will remove a source of mercury contamination to the environment. Additional studies at NIDBR have attempted to measure the concentrations of various forms of mercury residing in the dental wastewater, including ionic, organic and elemental mercury bound to particulate.

This is an important endeavor because different mercury species have different toxicity profiles and a meaningful assessment of mercury in dental wastewater must address the concentrations of all the different species present. Determining total mercury alone is not adequate to give a complete picture.

One of the questions you asked in your invitation to us was information on whether mercury solids methylate in sewer systems. In 1967, Swedish researchers demonstrated that bacteria are capable of transforming inorganic mercury into methylmercury, a more toxic and more readily absorbed form of the element. Many microorganisms, including bacteria and fungi, have been shown to possess the ability to methylate mercury.

NIDBR has been involved in the characterization of dental wastewater since 1993. We have measured total mercury and methylmercury levels in wastewater directly at the chair, from holding tanks and from sewers both upstream and downstream from dental treatment facilities. We found the percentage of methylmercury relative to total mercury to be a relatively small fraction. However, preliminary composite sampling of wastewater upstream and downstream from a large dental treatment facility showed a 12fold increase in total mercury leaving the dental clinic and a 3.6fold increase in methylmercury levels. One mile downstream from the clinic, the total mercury level had returned to the same as those upstream. However, the methylmercury level remains about 3.5fold higher than those upstream. The filter systems that we are installing in our dental clinics remove almost all of the total mercury prior to discharge into the waste stream.

Results of NIDBR studies underscore the importance of limiting the release of mercury into wastewater streams as the potential exists for mercury to be transformed into more toxic species.

That concludes my prepared remarks. We are ready for any questions you might have.

[The prepared statement of Captain Ragain follows:]

STATEMENT OF

CAPTAIN JAMES C. RAGAIN, JR, U. S. NAVY

NAVAL INSTITUTE FOR DENTAL AND BIOMEDICAL RESEARCH

(DENTAL CORPS)

BEFORE THE

SUBCOMMITTEE ON

HUMAN RIGHTS AND WELLNESS
OF THE
COMMITTEE ON GOVERNMENT REFORM

8 OCTOBER 2003

Mr. Chairman, Honorable Representatives, ladies and gentlemen, good afternoon. Thank you for inviting us to testify before the Subcommittee on Human Rights and Wellness. I am Captain James C. Ragain, Jr, Dental Corps, US Navy, Commanding Officer of the Naval Institute for Dental and Biomedical Research (NIDBR) located at the Naval Service Training Center, Great Lakes, Illinois. Accompanying me this afternoon are Commander John C. Kuehne, Dental Corps, US Navy, Head of the Bioenvironmental Sciences Department, and Dr. Mark E. Stone, Program Manager for the NIDBR Mercury Abatement Program.

NIDBR's research related to the control of mercury emissions from dental amalgam began in 1991 as a collaboration with the American Dental Association involving the evaluation of commercial amalgam separators. NIDBR instituted a Mercury Management Program to coordinate and direct the research efforts of a number of dental researchers and equipment specialists. This program made great strides in the design and installation of wastewater pretreatment systems at several Navy dental treatment facilities. NIDBR was then designated by Navy Dentistry as the Lead Agent for development, evaluation, and guidance regarding Navy-wide installation of wastewater pretreatment systems to minimize the environmental impact of Navy Dentistry. The tasking required that pretreatment systems be able to remove mercury in order to allow all Navy dental clinics to comply with local wastewater discharge standards. NIDBR was specifically tasked to assess current compliance of Dental Treatment Facilities (DTF), in meeting local discharge standards and to develop strategies to bring all DTFs in the Navy into compliance. This includes ships, field and mobile dental units.

In FY01, NIDBR began the implementation of a multi-year program to survey and install wastewater pretreatment systems in every Navy DTF worldwide. To date, pretreatment systems of various sizes have been successfully installed in 50% of all Navy dental clinics located within the continental United States. By the end of calendar year 2003, we expect to have completed the installation of mercury abatement systems in 95% of the Navy's US clinics. These systems meet local discharge limits, with anywhere from 95 to greater than 99% of total mercury removed from the wastewater. Previously completed wastewater characterization studies by NIDBR have enabled us to develop a pretreatment strategy that allows for the removal of mercury to extremely low levels, thus reducing mercury from grams per liter to micrograms per liter in the waste stream.

NIDBR's strategy involves the phased treatment of the dental-unit wastewater stream. Phase 1 is the removal of amalgam particulate through filtration and/or settling. Removal of particulate greater than 10 microns removes up to 95% of the total mercury in the waste stream. However, a significant amount of mercury is located in the dissolved or soluble fraction and is high enough to violate some local discharge limits. In Phase 2, the remaining dissolved mercury is driven to the ionic form by oxidation, and removed by sorbents.

This phased treatment program has proved very effective for both large and small dental treatment facilities. An additional benefit of the phased pretreatment strategy is the ability to deploy technology that can be scaled to meet variable local water treatment facilities' discharge limits.

Navy Dentistry's Mercury Abatement Program is a proactive effort intended to keep the Navy in compliance with local and overseas environmental requirements; and the successful implementation of these wastewater pretreatment systems will remove a source of mercury contamination to the environment.

Additional studies at NIDBR have attempted to measure the concentrations of various forms of mercury residing in the dental wastewater including ionic, organic and elemental mercury bound to particulate. This is an important endeavor because different mercury species have different toxicity profiles, and a meaningful assessment of mercury in dental wastewater must address the concentrations of all the different species present. Determining total mercury alone is not adequate to give a complete picture.

One of the questions you asked in your invitation to use was information on whether mercury solids methylate in sewer systems.

In 1967 Swedish researchers demonstrated that bacteria are capable of transforming inorganic mercury into methyl mercury, a more toxic and more readily absorbed form of the element. Many microorganisms, including bacteria and fungi, have been shown to possess the ability to methylate mercury.

NIDBR has been involved in the characterization of dental wastewater since 1993. We have measured total mercury and methyl mercury levels in wastewater, directly at the dental chair, from holding tanks, and from sewers both upstream and downstream from a dental treatment facility. We found the percentage of methyl mercury relative to total mercury to be a relatively small fraction; however, preliminary composite sampling of wastewater upstream and downstream from a large dental treatment facility showed a 12-fold increase in total mercury leaving the dental clinic and a 3.6-fold increase in methyl mercury levels. One mile downstream from the clinic, the total mercury level had returned to the same as those upstream. However, the methyl mercury level remains about 3-and-half-fold higher than those upstream. The filter systems that we are installing in our dental clinics remove almost all of the total mercury prior to discharge into the waste stream.

Results of NIDBR studies underscore the importance of limiting the release of mercury into wastewater streams, as the potential exists for mercury to be transformed into more toxic species.

That concludes my prepared remarks. We are ready for any questions you might have.

Mr. BURTON. Thank you, Captain. Mr. Cummings.

Mr. CUMMINGS. Thank you very much, Mr. Chairman. Mr. Chairman, Diane Watson, who is the ranking member on the committee, was not able to be here this afternoon because she is in her district. I just wanted to read her statement if that is OK with you, Mr. Chairman.

Thank you, Mr. Chairman. The Human Rights and Wellness hearing today is very important for the American people. This hearing will provide more information about the effects of elemental mercury and its use in dental fillings. In previous hearings we have discussed different aspects about the last remaining use of mercury inside the human body, but the environmental effects of mercury are equally disturbing.

Mercury is listed as the No. 1 environmental poison by the World Health Organization. The Environmental Protection Agency has listed mercury as No. 1 of the 19 most persistent and bio-accumulative toxic metals. Last Thursday, October 2, 2003, Ballou Senior High School was shut down in Southeast Washington, DC, due to 250 milliliters, or approximately 450 fillings worth of mercury. I understand the public concern over the mercury spill, but we should also be concerned with approximately one-half gram of the same hazardous material being placed in the mouths of our children and adults in each amalgam filling.

In a recent report entitled "Dentists the Menace," dentists were called the biggest mercury polluters in the United States. Consider these facts. Dentistry is one of the only unregulated major sources of mercury discharges to the environment. Dental fillings constitute the largest source of direct mercury pollution in wastewater. Dentistry is the fifth largest consumer of mercury in the United States. And dentists use toxic mercury in silver fillings which are made of 43 to 54 percent mercury.

Dentists improperly dispose of mercury dental fillings every day. Mercury dental fillings are put in the trash that eventually will be incinerated, releasing poisonous gases and vapors into the air. Properly cremated loved ones release the same mercury contaminants into the air through mercury fillings. Dentists also discard mercury dental fillings by putting them in landfills, contaminating the soil and surrounding water sources. Mercury dental fillings pose too much risk for not only the health of dental patients but environmental and agricultural safety.

Mercury is constantly being discharged into our environment, polluting our water sources. The body tissue of fish easily absorbs mercury suspended in water. Ultimately we eat this toxic mercury. Pregnant women are constantly being warned not to eat shark, swordfish or mackerel due to their extremely high accumulation of mercury. If they are warned not to eat fish, why are they not constantly being warned to not use mercury dental fillings?

That is the statement of Ms. Watson, Mr. Chairman. I thank you for allowing me to put that into the record.

[The prepared statement of Hon. Elijah E. Cummings follows:]

Elijah E. Cummings (signature)

Subcommittee on Human Rights and Wellness
Hearing on "The Environmental Impact of Mercury-Containing Dental Amalgams"
Congressman Elijah Cummings
October 8, 2003

Mr. Chairman:

Thank you for convening today's hearing to discuss the environmental impact of mercury in dental amalgams. In this ongoing series of hearings, the Committee has also investigated mercury-containing thimerosal in vaccines, and mercury-containing amalgams. During those hearings, we learned that a variety of developmental and neurological disorders could directly be linked to mercury in the human body.

Another frightening piece of information that we learned during those hearings is that other sources of mercury in the human body are water and certain foods, specifically fish. As I stated, this is frightening and an issue of significant concern. So much so that the Environmental Protection Agency (EPA) and various state and local environmental agencies around the country have issued advisories against eating fish from specific lakes and streams. Furthermore, the scientific evidence supporting such advisories is abundant.

This leads us to the chain reaction contamination of lakes, rivers, and streams with mercury discharge from dental offices. I say chain reaction because once dental office discharge is released into municipal sewer systems, its natural progression leads back to nature where it enters the food chain to be absorbed

1   by humans. Therein lies the problem; the human body is not designed to

2   eliminate mercury once it is ingested. Unfortunately, mercury in the body

3   accumulates in vital organs such as the brain.

4

5   I am glad to see that one of our distinguished witnesses is from the Association

6   of Metropolitan Sewerage Agencies (AMSA). Mr. Hornbeck, one of several

7   studies done by your agency reported that mercury levels in household

8   wastewater were sufficiently high to pose Clean Water Act compliance

9   problems for the nation's wastewater treatment plants. A subsequent report

10   revealed that the consumption of fish from waters contaminated with mercury

11   offers the greatest risk of exposure to the contaminant. I know that your

12   agency has taken a proactive position in identifying problems and

13   recommending a national strategy to reduce mercury in the environment. I

14   will save my questions regarding progress in that area for later.

15

16   Although many scientists believe that dental mercury accounts for a small

17   percentage of the total mercury problem, it remains a significant source of

18   contamination through wastewater treatment plants.   I find this upsetting

19   due to the fact that there are options to the use of dental amalgams.   One

20   example is the use by pediatric dentists of plastic FDA approved tooth-colored

21   materials that are bonded to the teeth, thereby eliminating the need for

22   amalgams.

23

24   Mr. Chairman, as you well know, mercury is one of the most toxic minerals

25   found in nature, second only to radioactive materials. Whether the risks of

26   mercury contamination are thought to be minor or significant, I feel that

27   eliminating it as a health hazard is our goal. I welcome our distinguished

1 witness and look forward to our discussion on reducing and ultimately
2 eliminating negative environment impacts of mercury-containing dental
3 amalgams.

Mr. BURTON. No problem. Thank you.

First of all, I want to commend the Navy for its constructive actions that they have taken to reduce dental mercury in their facilities around the world. Captain, you didn't mention in your testimony why the Navy first got interested in mercury abatement. Wasn't there a particularly alarming and costly incident involving the naval dental clinic in the Virginia Beach-Hampton Roads area?

Captain RAGAIN. Yes, sir, there was.

Mr. BURTON. Do you want to go into that in detail or do you want me just to read what happened?

Captain RAGAIN. It is up to you, Mr. Chairman.

Mr. BURTON. Well, the answer is the Hampton Roads sewage treatment plant finally refused to accept the Navy's sewage because it contained too much mercury. The Navy had to dump their wastewater into 55-gallon drums and then have them hauled away by a hazardous materials company that charged $900 per barrel. Why did that happen?

Captain RAGAIN. Why did it? I don't understand your question.

Mr. BURTON. Why would that sewage treatment plant not accept the refuse from your facility?

Captain RAGAIN. I wouldn't know, sir.

Mr. BURTON. Well, they said it was because there was too much mercury going in there, isn't that correct?

Captain RAGAIN. I haven't talked to that plant, sir. I don't know.

Mr. BURTON. Well, you do know that they wouldn't accept that, don't you?

Captain RAGAIN. That was their statement, sir.

Mr. BURTON. Captain, come on now. You don't know about this? You don't know what happened?

Captain RAGAIN. I know that we were required to put our dental wastewater in cans because the discharge limits exceeded the local PWC limits.

Mr. BURTON. And the reason for that was?

Captain RAGAIN. Because of the discharge of the water. Not why they wouldn't accept the cans.

Mr. BURTON. What was in the water? It was mercury, wasn't it?

Captain RAGAIN. The mercury had spiked, yes, sir.

Mr. BURTON. Yes. Now, the mercury is being removed because of the amalgam separators and 95 to 90 percent of the mercury is now being removed, is that right?

Captain RAGAIN. Yes, sir.

Mr. BURTON. Let me ask you both a question. If mercury is unsafe before it is put into your teeth and it is unsafe afterwards because it has to be collected and handled very carefully, why is it safe in your mouth? How about you, Mr. Grubbs?

Mr. GRUBBS. To be honest, I am not sure I can answer that one either, sir. The jurisdiction for EPA deals with pollution into the environment from sewage treatment plants, into the air, and so forth. With regard to exposure to the body, my understanding is that is Food and Drug Administration where those decisions are made. So I have not looked at that specific question.

Mr. BURTON. The FDA. How about you, Captain?

Captain RAGAIN. When it is in the mouth, it is bound into the amalgam and it is not released.

Mr. BURTON. Let's followup on that. We had a scientist here—we had scientists, more than one here, who said that they had tested amalgams in a glass of water and checked them and they were releasing mercury even though they were supposed to be inert in that filling. They had done several tests to show that was occurring. They also showed when heat was applied or cold was applied that vapors were emitted from the fillings that showed that the mercury was being released.

When a filling is taken out and it is put into the sewage of the office, let's say a dentist flushes it down the drain like a lot of them have been known to do, why is that a danger if it is inert in the mouth? If it is hard in the mouth and it is safe because it has that other residue with it, you know, when they make the filling, why is it not safe when it leaves the mouth?

Captain RAGAIN. Sir, I'm going to defer that question, if I may, to Commander Kuehne. He is a materials expert in the bioenvironmental area and he probably could have a better answer there that you are looking for.

Mr. BURTON. Sure.

Commander KUEHNE. Thank you, sir.

First of all, I would say it is not really my decision to rule definitively on what is or isn't safe. The scientific panels that have met in the past to evaluate amalgam as a material have deemed it to be a safe and effective material.

However, to answer your question, the real issue is that when the amalgam is in the waste stream or in the environment, for as long as it remains there, which is indefinite, it is subject to bacterial conversion, bacterial organisms in the environment that convert the source of mercury in the amalgam to methylmercury.

Mr. BURTON. You really believe that is how it happens? The bacteria in your mouth doesn't have any effect?

Commander KUEHNE. I don't know, sir. I wouldn't say that it's impossible. All I can say is that the scientific evidence to date that I am aware of have not shown any significant release of free mercury or methylmercury from fillings in the mouth.

Mr. BURTON. Have you heard of Dr. Boyd Haley?

Commander KUEHNE. No, sir.

Mr. BURTON. You haven't had any conversations with him? Dr. Haley testified before our committee, and Dr. Haley went into great detail. He is a biological scientist.

Mr. ROWE. Yes, and he is Chair of the Department of Chemistry.

Mr. BURTON. He is the chairman of the Department of Chemistry down there at the University of Kentucky.

He has done an enormous amount of research on this. He says there is absolutely no doubt, no doubt whatsoever that the mercury fillings in the mouth and afterwards does emit vapors that get into the blood stream, mercury vapors, and can cause neurological problems and that when you chew every once in a while you might chew a hard substance and it breaks off and gets into your system, it can also cause some damage. You wouldn't argue with that, though?

Commander KUEHNE. Sir, again, I wouldn't say that it is impossible. I'm just saying that all of the scientific evidence and the panels that have met in the past, NIH panels and other panels that have come together to weigh all the scientific evidence that is available, have so far concluded that there is no significant release of toxic mercury from fillings that are placed in the mouth.

Mr. BURTON. When I was a little boy, we used to find old thermometers, and we would break them, and we would do this with the mercury. You know what I'm talking about, when you were kids? I wonder why they don't do that anymore? Because we found out that the mercury was toxic, and it could really cause severe damage. In my district, we spilled a very small amount of it, and they evacuated two neighborhoods, had people come in, looked like they were from outer space to clean it up. That happened in this school here in Washington, DC. Yet we continue to put mercury in our mouths. Would you swallow a mercury amalgam? You would swallow it? You wouldn't worry about it?

Commander KUEHNE. Yes, sir. Honestly myself, because of what I know about the differences between the absorption of elemental mercury vapor through the lungs and solid amalgam absorption through the gut, it personally wouldn't bother me. I would much rather swallow a dental amalgam than to breathe in the same amount of mercury vapor. I would be very worried about breathing in the same amount.

Mr. BURTON. If you knew it was being emitted from your teeth? If you knew that vapor was being emitted——

Commander KUEHNE. Yes, sir. Again, I'm not trying to defend it. I'm not trying to say it is impossible. All I am trying to say is, from what I know of the scientific evidence to date—I have dental amalgams in my mouth. I am not worried about the emission of mercury. I do know that elemental mercury vapor is toxic and easily absorbed into the body. I do know that amalgam has the potential to methylate in the environment. So both of those issues I am concerned about, and we are taking action for it.

Mr. BURTON. I am going to yield to Mr. Cummings, but just let me tell you that there is a machine that my dentist used to show the amount of mercury vapor that was being emitted from the amalgams I had in my mouth. It has been pretty much proved that this machine is accurate. I don't know if you guys have any mercury fillings in your mouth, but we happen to have one of those machines over there if you would like to check it out before you leave. It might be a very intellectually stimulating experience for you.

Captain RAGAIN. I've got five in my mouth.

Mr. BURTON. You have five in your mouth?

Captain RAGAIN. Yes, sir.

Mr. BURTON. You might want to check that out before you leave. It might make you want to get them out of there.

Mr. Cummings.

Mr. CUMMINGS. Just a few questions, Mr. Chairman.

Commander Kuehne, you had said with regard to the amalgam and the mercury in the filling that you did not believe a significant amount of mercury was released. What do you consider not significant, or significant?

Commander KUEHNE. That is a good question. I guess that is what it comes down to, I think, because almost everything could have some trace mercury concentration if you could employ methods fine enough to detect it. I would say for myself as a standard compared to the amount I would get in a normal diet. In other words, I think that whatever mercury would be released from fillings in my mouth would be insignificant when you compared it to a normal diet. If I would try to exclude the same amount of mercury from my diet completely, I would probably have to eliminate most if not all of the things I ate. It is a naturally occurring element in the Earth's crust. It is present in many foods, not just fish.

Mr. CUMMINGS. A woman who is pregnant, is she more susceptible to harm from mercury?

Commander KUEHNE. Sir, with all due respect, I can understand why you would be asking us this, but really I think these are questions that the FDA and WHO and people like that have—it is in their purview to rule on those things. WHO and FDA, organizations like that.

Mr. CUMMINGS. I understand that. Just based upon your knowledge—and I understand and I am not trying to take you out of your realm, but I am just asking you a general question. You make decisions, you have to address these issues, and I am sure you have some general knowledge of what you believe. If you do, that is all I am asking you. I am not trying to put you in a corner or anything like that. So you do believe that a woman—in other words, you would not like to see a woman who is pregnant absorbing mercury, swallowing it from her teeth or anything, I take it?

Commander KUEHNE. First of all, I would be concerned about, or I would advise a pregnant woman to exercise some caution, educate herself about the dangers of mercury consumption. I think the place to begin with that personally would not be with the fillings in her mouth if they are already there. I think the place to begin would be looking at the diet, fish consumption, to know where the fish comes from and the concentration of mercury that would be in the fish, water, the things that would be consumed on a regular basis daily. I would never try to argue that absolutely zero amount—there may be very small amounts of mercury that would be released from whatever fillings she would have in her mouth, but, again, I think that in terms of her total dietary consumption that would not be my major concern.

Mr. CUMMINGS. A filling—when a person—sometimes a doctor will tell you, a dentist will say, we've got to give you another filling. I am just wondering, is that—I mean, something has happened to cause the filling that you had not to be doing what it was doing before. There is some kind of problem.

Captain RAGAIN. It depends on the clinical situation.

Mr. CUMMINGS. So I guess what I am getting at is that if there is—if something has happened to that filling, and that is assuming there is some still there, would you assume that there is a release of mercury that is higher than the insignificant or amount that you just talked about? Are you following what I am saying?

Commander KUEHNE. Yes, sir.

Mr. CUMMINGS. I mean, it happens all the time. People go to the dentist. The dentist says, look, we've got to refill this. I was just curious.

Commander KUEHNE. Yes, sir. Again, we're getting into an area that may be as much opinion or judgment call as anything else, but, in my own judgment, it is not actually the amount of mercury that would be released during normal chewing that would be a concern. But when you either place or remove the mercury, the patient exposure to mercury at that time would be higher than once it is placed and set. So in the placement and the removal process that is when proper practices should be followed in order to minimize that risk exposure to the patient and the dentist, their staff, as well as to the environment.

Dentists do and should follow certain procedures that we, for instance, would use in a rubber dam which protects the patient but provides a barrier between the patient and the removal using high-speed suction. If the proper filters to remove mercury are attached to that suction, you can do that procedure safely or you can do that procedure where it represents a larger risk to the patient and the environment.

Mr. CUMMINGS. Finally, Mr. Chairman, from an environmental standpoint, what is the safest way to get rid of, I guess it would be, mercury waste? What is the safest way to do that? In other words, so that you minimize any kind of harm to the environment, what is the ideal way to do that?

Commander KUEHNE. First of all, to remove all of it from the wastewater before—again in my opinion, it would be to first of all remove all of it from the wastewater before it is sent to the treatment facility plant, to collect it and dry it so that it is in a dry amalgam form. The dissolved portion of the mercury, which would be ionic mercury, that would be dissolved in water. We use a process that binds that ionic mercury to a resin, and it is chemically bound at that point, and at that point it won't be released from that chemical bond.

Then to collect that in those states, the dry particulate amalgam and the chemical resin, all the forms of mercury that you have used to remove it and to send that to a licensed recycler or a company that is licensed and knows how to reclaim that mercury or dispose of it properly.

Mr. CUMMINGS. So a small amount of mercury can do some serious damage? I mean, the chairman just talked about—we had the school to close and then the chairman talked about a small amount—were you talking about in your district?

Mr. BURTON. Yes.

Mr. CUMMINGS. It can do a lot. I assume this is something that sends off a lot of red lights. I guess that is why we are here.

Commander KUEHNE. The risk, that is really a difficult question to answer. When you say a small amount and a lot of damage, those are terms that are difficult to quantify from a scientific point of view. And it really represents what somebody would consider small, what——

Mr. CUMMINGS. I will let the chairman—because he knows what happened in his district or wherever. I guess what I am trying to do is make sure I get a real clear picture of exactly how much of this substance would cause any reasonable health official or provider to be alarmed.

Commander KUEHNE. I wouldn't want to breathe mercury vapor on a regular basis over a long period of time, because mercury vapor is well absorbed across the lungs, it accumulates in the body and it has long-term health effects. So I certainly—a small amount of mercury vapor like that, what was released in the school, especially if it is inhaled chronically over a long period of time certainly represents a health risk. A consistent ingestion of methylmercury from fish or organic tissue, once it is taken up in the food chain, especially by more susceptible people like pregnant women, again over a long period of time, certainly represents a definite health risk. But in both of those cases you have to consider the form that the mercury is in, whether it is in elemental mercury, liquid, vapor state, whether it is amalgam, whether it is methylmercury in the organic tissue of fish. Each one of those things represents a different situation. The way it is ingested represents—the time of exposure, whether it is a one-time exposure.

It is like x-rays. Being out in the sun for 5 minutes represents a different risk than being out in the sun for 3 hours. It depends on the angle of the sun.

To say absolutely mercury in every form, in every condition, in every concentration is a huge risk, no, sir, I couldn't go that far. But it definitely is a health risk.

Captain RAGAIN. It is like chlorine, chlorine gas. It is very toxic, but we have all had sodium chloride today in salt.

Mr. CUMMINGS. Thank you, Mr. Chairman.

Mr. BURTON. Mercury is supposedly one of the most toxic if not the most toxic substances around, isn't it? Is that not correct, when it is ingested? Incidentally, where did you get all this information? Commander, where did you get all this information?

Commander KUEHNE. All the information about mercury?

Mr. BURTON. About mercury. Do you have a degree in that? Have you studied it? Are you a chemist?

Commander KUEHNE. Yes, sir. I'm a dentist. We studied it in dental school. I have a master's degree in dental materials and being involved with research for a number of years. I have read research papers, and I guess that is where I get my information from.

Mr. BURTON. You have never read any research papers from the University of Kentucky and the head of their chemistry department down there that has worked on this?

Mr. STONE. I think most of the literature that we're familiar with is related to the environmental exposure to it, to the mercury. I think a lot of the issues you are talking about are exposure to humans, related to human health effects. We're sort of on the other side of that with the wastewater issue.

Mr. BURTON. Well, the fact of the matter is the wastewater treatment people of this country say that the amalgams getting into the wastewater treatment system has caused an awful lot of problems, correct?

Commander KUEHNE. Yes.

Mr. BURTON. And it wouldn't be in the wastewater treatment system if we didn't have mercury in our mouths in the first place, would it? It wouldn't be getting in there from the amalgams if it wasn't in our mouths, isn't that correct?

Commander KUEHNE. Yes, sir.

Mr. BURTON. What I can't understand is if there is a risk to our health, either before it is in our mouths, after it is in our mouths, while it is in our mouths, we know that once it gets into the food chain it is a real problem and there is an increasing number of items in our food chain, you mentioned fish, that are becoming a real problem as far as human beings consuming them.

One of the ways they are getting that is from the water that goes through the wastewater treatment system into our lakes and our streams around this country. It seems to me that we would want to get that out of there, especially if there is an alternative substance that can be used to fill teeth. Why would you use something that you knew was toxic if you knew there was something else? Because it is less expensive is the answer. But the fact of the matter is there are ways to deal with this without putting mercury in people's teeth.

The other thing that is very interesting is when they put mercury fillings in your mouth, they aren't inert while they are putting them in your mouth. They mix them up. The person who is mixing them up has some exposure, I would imagine, from mixing them on a regular basis. Then they put it into some kind of a syringe-type thing and they jam it down into your tooth, into the cavity that they have exposed by drilling. And when they jam it down into your tooth, I know that parts of it fall down into your mouth, parts of it, and it is not yet inert, it is still liquid, because they say, oh, you've got to wait about 5 minutes before we take this brace off that holds it in place. And that inert material, that material that is not yet inert, is ingested into your body, because I have swallowed part of it because I couldn't get it all out when I rinsed after they put the filling in. Are you telling me that none of that is dangerous? It is not yet inert. It is still in the syringe. He puts it in your mouth. Are you saying there is no danger there?

Commander KUEHNE. No, sir. I certainly don't say there is no danger. I think—it is just—we recognize—I think what we are here to agree to is that we recognize the long-term consequences of putting amalgam waste into the environment and that is why the Navy has taken steps to stop that. Beyond that, what constitutes an acceptable risk——

Mr. BURTON. So there is a risk.

Commander KUEHNE. There is a risk in every activity that I can think of. And certainly there is a risk of—there are many risks associated with the practice of dentistry.

Mr. BURTON. You don't need to go any further. The fact of the matter is there is a risk, and you think it is an acceptable risk to put an amalgam in people's mouths. There is a divergence of opinion on that subject. We have had scientists who say they have tested it very thoroughly over many years, and there are vapors that escape into people's mouths. There are also chips and so forth that fall into the body. If there is a biological thing that takes place, you said that there is some bacteria that might eat away at one of these amalgams and cause a release of the mercury. It could happen in our bodies as well. But the fact of the matter is there is a risk, and I do appreciate that.

Do any of you have any final comments you would like to make?

Captain RAGAIN. No, sir.

Mr. GRUBBS. No, sir.

Mr. BURTON. Thank you very much. We appreciate it.

Our next panel is Dr. Frederick Eichmiller, director, American Dental Association Health Foundation; Mr. Norman LeBlanc, chief, Technical Services at the Hampton Roads Sanitation District; Mr. Peter Berglund, principal engineer at the Metropolitan Council of Environmental Services; and Mr. David Galvin, project manager, Hazardous Waste Management Program at the King County Department of Natural Resources.

Would you all please stand?

I appreciate you sticking around to hear what they have to say. [Witnesses sworn.]

Mr. BURTON. Since there are a large number of you and it is getting a little late and I apologize for that, if we could keep our comments to around 5 minutes, I would really appreciate it. We will put the rest of your statements in the record.

Dr. Eichmiller.

STATEMENTS OF DR. FREDRICK EICHMILLER, DIRECTOR, AMERICAN DENTAL ASSOCIATION HEALTH FOUNDATION, PAFFENBARGER RESEARCH CENTER, NATIONAL BUREAU OF STANDARDS & TECHNOLOGY, ACCOMPANIED BY JEROME BOWMAN, ADA STAFF ATTORNEY; NORMAN LEBLANC, CHIEF, TECHNICAL SERVICES, HAMPTON ROADS SANITATION DISTRICT; PETER BERGLUND, PE, PRINCIPAL ENGINEER, METROPOLITAN COUNCIL OF ENVIRONMENTAL SERVICES, INDUSTRIAL WASTE SECTION; AND DAVID GALVIN, PROJECT MANAGER, HAZARDOUS WASTE MANAGEMENT PROGRAM, KING COUNTY DEPARTMENT OF NATURAL RESOURCES AND PARKS, WATER AND LAND RESOURCES DIVISION

Dr. EICHMILLER. Mr. Chairman, members of the committee, my name is Fred Eichmiller. I am a dentist and director of the Paffenbarger Research Center, one of the world's premier dental research facilities, an affiliate of the ADA Health Foundation in Gaithersburg, MD. Scientists at the Paffenbarger Center conduct basic and applied studies to improve the science and art of dentistry and benefit the health of the American public.

With me today is Mr. Jerome Bowman, an ADA staff attorney who has been involved in the Association's efforts to forge a partnership with the EPA to further minimize the environmental impact of waste dental amalgam.

I speak today on behalf of the ADA's members, 147,000 individual dentists and their families who live in the same communities and consume the same water as everyone else.

The ADA bases its policy positions on the best available scientific evidence, so in crafting its best management practices and a national advocacy plan to reduce amalgam waste discharge we sought first to expand and improve the scientific data available on the amount of waste amalgam that dental offices actually discharge and what happens to any amalgam that is discharged. To that end, we commissioned ENVIRON to conduct a scientific assessment. The author of that assessment, Mr. Jay Vandeven, is with us here today and available to answer any questions or any additional questions that Mr. Bowman and I cannot answer.

I will note that because mercury in dental amalgam is bound as a stable ally with other metals, the studies thus far indicate that very little of it dissolves to become bioavailable. In other words, even when amalgam enters the wastewater, mercury from amalgam is unlikely to enter the food chain.

Despite this, we asked that the ENVIRON assessment ignore that premise. The data it reports and the conclusions it reaches reflect a worst-case assumption that all of the mercury in any waste amalgam could eventually become bioavailable.

The key findings of that study include the contribution of mercury in surface waters and sludge that are attributed to dental offices is far worse than those from other sources. The chairside traps and vacuum pump filters capture approximately 77 percent of the amalgam discharged in wastewater by dental offices. Amalgam separators when used in conjunction with best management practices can capture up to 95 percent of the amalgam not captured by the traps and filters. However, because public water treatment facilities capture 95 percent or more of that same material, the use of separators ultimately would have little impact on the level of mercury in the surface water or fish.

The ENVIRON report underwent prepublication review by individuals from AMSA and the EPA.

Let me make it clear that the ADA does not see the ENVIRON report as justification for inaction on amalgam waste. Rather, the Association is using the report's findings to guide the process of enhancing our longstanding commitment to foster an environmentally sound dental practice.

Based on the ENVIRON findings, the Association this year published best management practices for amalgam waste to provide its members with comprehensive, easy-to-follow recommendations for managing the waste and finding a recycler. Our goal is 100 percent recycling of amalgam waste captured by dental offices.

The ADA recognizes amalgam separators as a potentially valuable adjunct to a dental office's waste management procedures in situations where environmental concerns or local law warrant them. However, the Association believes that the decision about whether to use separators should be made on a case-by-case basis in response to local needs and within the context of comprehensive best management practices. In fact, many State dental associations have reached or are currently working on agreements with their State environmental authorities, and many of these agreements involve the voluntary use of amalgam separators.

The ADA has and will continue to publish and otherwise disseminate useful information for dentists who want or need to install separators, including seminars at major dental meetings and articles in the peer-reviewed Journal of the American Dental Association, which is sent to all of our members.

Finally, I will note that the ADA is actively engaged in discussions with the EPA with the aim of establishing a national partnership to help State and local authorities develop sensible policies regarding dental amalgam waste. These could include recycling, collection programs, best management practices and other common-sense measures.

Mr. Chairman, that concludes my statement, but I respectfully request just a moment more of your time to read the text of the resolutions that are going before our House of Delegates and will be considered in 2 weeks at that meeting. I believe these actions give good testimony to the ADA's commitment to environmentally sound dental practice.

The first resolution is, resolved that the Association strongly encourages dentists to adhere to best management practice and supports other voluntary efforts by dentists to reduce amalgam discharges in dental office wastewater.

Be it further resolved that the Association encourages constituent and component societies to enter into collaborative arrangements with regional, State or local wastewater authorities to address their concerns about amalgam in dental office wastewater.

Be it further resolved that the appropriate agencies of the Association continue to disseminate information to the constituent and component societies to help them address concerns of regional, State or local wastewater authorities about amalgam in dental office wastewater.

Be it further resolved that the appropriate agencies of the Association continue to investigate products and services that will help dentists effectively reduce amalgam in dental office wastewater and keep the profession advised.

Be it further resolved that the Association include in its advocacy messages the importance of basing environmental regulations or guidances affecting dental offices on sound science.

And be it further resolved that the Association continue to identify and urge the Environmental Protection Agency to fund studies that accurately and appropriately identify whether amalgam wastewater discharge affects the environment.

Thank you for allowing us to appear before this panel. We will be glad to answer your questions.

Mr. BURTON. That resolution you are talking about is not mandatory, though, is it? It is voluntary?

Dr. EICHMILLER. Yes, it is voluntary.

Mr. BURTON. Thank you.

[The prepared statement of Dr. Eichmiller follows:]

STATEMENT OF THE
AMERICAN DENTAL ASSOCIATION

TO THE

WELLNESS AND HUMAN RIGHTS SUBCOMMITTEE
GOVERNMENT REFORM COMMITTEE

UNITED STATES HOUSE OF REPRESENTATIVES

ON

THE ENVIRONMENTAL IMPACT OF MERCURY-CONTAINING
DENTAL AMALGAM

SUBMITTED BY

FREDERICK C. EICHMILLER, D.D.S.

OCTOBER 8, 2003

Thank you, Mr. Chairman and members of the Subcommittee on Human Rights & Wellness for the opportunity to testify today on behalf of the American Dental Association (ADA) concerning "The Environmental Impact of Mercury-Containing Dental Amalgam." The ADA represents over 70 percent of the dentists in the United States. My name is Dr. Frederick C. Eichmiller. I am the director of the ADA Foundation's Paffenbarger Research Center in Gaithersburg, Maryland. With me is Mr. Jerome Bowman, an attorney in the ADA's legal division. Mr. Bowman has been involved in the efforts of the ADA to forge a partnership with the Environmental Protection Agency (EPA) to further minimize the impact on the environment of waste dental amalgam.

I speak today on behalf of ADA members, 147,000 individual dentists and their families who live in the same communities and consume the same water as everyone else. We're committed—both as health professionals and as individuals who depend on a clean, safe environment—to responsible stewardship of our natural resources. Protecting the public's health through appropriate handling and disposal of dental waste is a natural extension of our top priority—to provide the best possible oral health care to patients.

Evaluation of Mercury in Dental Facility Wastewater

I have been asked to talk today primarily about the scientific assessment that the ADA commissioned from ENVIRON International Corporation concerning the release of mercury from dental facilities. The author of that assessment, Mr. Jay Vandeven, is in the audience should the panel have questions that I cannot answer.

The ENVIRON report, "Assessment of Mercury in the Form of Amalgam in Dental Wastewater in the United States," (August 12, 2003) uses a "materials balance approach" to calculate the average discharge of mercury from a dental office and its aggregate impact on wastewater treatment plants.

The materials balance approach uses survey data on the number and frequency of amalgam restorations and a critical review of the scientific literature on the discharge of amalgam from dental offices. The results are compared to the known aggregate sale of amalgam and the cumulative data on mercury concentration in effluent leaving wastewater treatment plants and in sewerage sludge, as well as other measured ambient concentrations of mercury. The materials balance approach acknowledges that the amount of dental amalgam discharged cannot be more than dental amalgam used and avoids the variability inherent in sampling an episodic discharge using only a handful of measurements to represent the over 100,000 dental offices nationwide.

Dentistry, as a science-based profession, bases its positions on matters of public policy on the best available scientific evidence. This is why the ADA based its comprehensive plan to address amalgam discharges from dental offices on a scientific assessment of environmental impact. A key consideration for dentists, as small business people and health care providers, must be to use limited financial resources in a way that will best promote patient care, enhance the safety of the dental office **and** protect the environment. We considered it important, therefore, to include a cost-benefit analysis in the ENVIRON study.

To summarize, briefly, the key findings of the ENVIRON study are:

- The ENVIRON study calculated that: (1) about 35 tons of mercury is used each year by dentists; (2) about 29.7 tons goes down the drain in the office sinks; (3) about 23.2 tons are captured by chair side traps and vacuum filter systems; (4) about 6.5 tons of total mercury enters POTWs from dental offices; but (5) only 0.3 tons is discharged to the surface water bodies and another 0.1 tons enters surface water from air emissions of sludge incinerators. Because of the decrease in industrial use of mercury, approximately 35% to 45% of the mercury entering POTWs is from dental office sources, but these sources do not significantly contribute to the mercury levels in surface water because, according to EPA, the "principal sources of fish contamination" with mercury "are air emissions of mercury from coal burning power plants, municipal waste incinerators and other industrial sources." US EPA, Star Report, Vol. 4, Issue 1, Mercury Transport and Fate in Watersheds at 2 (October 2000).

- The primary source of total mercury in surface water and fish is air deposition, not water discharges. (See Table 1, attached) Consequently, even if all dental amalgam were completely eliminated from wastewater, it would not significantly reduce the levels of mercury in fish and surface water. (See Table 2, attached)

- The chair-side trap and vacuum pump filter commonly used in dental offices is effective in capturing approximately 77 percent of the amalgam discharged in wastewater by dental offices.

- Because the mercury in dental amalgam is tightly bound and is released primarily as particulates, most of the amalgam (95%) that is not already captured by dental office traps and vacuums is captured in the sewage treatment plants.

- Amalgam separators, when used in conjunction with BMPs, will capture up to 95% of the remaining 23% not captured by the traps and filters. This results in a 33% to 43% reduction in mercury influent to POTWs due to the use of amalgam separators. But, because of the efficiencies of the POTW systems (capturing 95% of the amalgam entering the system), the incremental amount of amalgam captured by an amalgam separator will have little impact on the level of methylmercury in surface water or, more importantly, in fish. The Scientific Assessment compared the effectiveness of amalgam separators in achieving EPA's regulatory goal (reducing the methylmercury levels in fish to 0.3 ppm or lower) utilizing the analytical tools that EPA consistently uses when it decides whether potential pollution control measure is warranted or whether one method is preferable to another (i.e., cost-effectiveness). This comparison indicates that using amalgam separators is much more costly per ton of mercury than the level EPA has determined does not warrant further controls for major industries. In fact, the cost per ton is higher than EPA guidance recommends for releases of mercury to the Great Lakes. The ADA believes that many local factors need to be considered in deciding which mercury sources should be addressed, the timing of such efforts, and the most appropriate mercury reduction measure appropriate for each type of source. Thus, no one rule can be applied to all dental offices. (See Table 3, attached)

ENVIRON subjected the study to pre-publication review from the Association of Metropolitan Sewerage Agencies (AMSA) and the EPA. Based on their input, ENVIRON made some modifications, but none affect the essential conclusion that discharges of dental amalgam in dental office wastewater do not contribute significantly to mercury in the environment. The ENVIRON study was submitted to both internal peer review (i.e. within the ADA and state dental associations) and external peer review by sewage treatment authorities and EPA reviews. The study will be submitted for publication soon and is expected to be published next year.

The ENVIRON report demonstrates that much can be achieved through the conscientious use of best management practices to capture and recycle amalgam waste. As a matter of public policy, the only reasonable approach is a case-by-case evaluation to determine whether additional amalgam capture technology, such as installation of amalgam separators, is necessary. We believe that where the local environmental conditions (i.e. mercury levels in surface waters, sludge, sediment or fish) do not exceed regulatory limits, stringent controls on mercury releases from dental offices should not be required. Where the concentrations of mercury in surface water, municipal sludge, sediment or fish tissue do exceed regulatory limits, dental offices are willing to do their fair share and to voluntarily go beyond BMPs to help in reducing the release of mercury in the form of dental amalgam.

Best Management Practices

For more than 25 years, the ADA has encouraged proper handling of amalgam to prevent its release into the environment. Last year, based on the findings of the ENVIRON study, the ADA strengthened its recommendations and increased its educational efforts aimed at dentists. The ADA "Best Management Practices for Amalgam Waste" (ADA BMPs) published in February 2003 provide comprehensive, easy-to-follow recommendations for managing amalgam waste and finding a recycler. They continue the ADA's strong recommendation that dentists use only precapsulated amalgam alloy to avoid the release of free mercury.

Our goal is 100 percent recycling of amalgam waste captured by dental offices.

The ADA's 2003 BMPs for Amalgam Waste makes it clear that although mercury in the form of dental amalgam is very stable, amalgam should not be disposed of in the garbage, infectious waste "red bag", or sharps container. Dental amalgam waste should also not be rinsed down the drain. The goal is to keep amalgam waste separate so it can be safely recycled. The Association is making a sustained effort to disseminate the BMP criteria to all of our members and has promoted the new BMPs in ADA publications and our web page.

In fact, the ADA will host a booth at the ADA Annual Session later this month with the theme -- "Protecting the Environment: What the Dental Office Can Do." The booth will offer useful information on practices, products and services to help manage dental office wastes. Visitors can learn the latest information on the ADA's best management practices for amalgam waste, managing silver and lead waste and recycling information as well as see a variety of amalgam separators, get information on the different types of available separator technologies and learn what to consider when purchasing a separator.

In addition, the ADA will host an open session course on dental office wastewater management at the Annual Session to discuss "Dental Office Water Quality and Wastewater Management." This program will include:

- an overview of the sources of mercury to the environment,
- a review of regulatory requirements and trends for mercury control,
- a discussion of ADA-approved best management practices for mercury waste streams, and
- a review of available amalgam separator technologies, installation, operational requirements and recycling options.

As noted above, dentists share the concerns of the vast majority of Americans that we should all take reasonable steps to ensure that our environment is protected. The ADA will continue to actively educate our members on the benefits of universal adherence to BMPs.

Dental Amalgam Separators

The ADA does not oppose the use of dental amalgam separators by dentists. In fact, the ADA is the primary source of information to help dentists who wish to install a separator find the right equipment. We recognize that there may well be specific environmental conditions or local laws that would make the use of separators appropriate. For example, where local environmental conditions demonstrate that environmental standards are exceeded and airborne sources of mercury are not predominant, separators may make sense.

However, local environmental conditions vary widely. A requirement to install separators in dental offices throughout the country is not justified. One size does not fit all. One problem with universal separator requirements is that such requirements do little to protect the environment. Separators and Publicly Owned Treatment Works (POTWs) remove very nearly the same size amalgam particles. In other words, separators offer little additional protection to the environment. Thus, where significant surface water contamination is due to air deposition, separators simply will not make much difference, or do much to solve the problem of surface water contamination. Where air deposition is not a significant source of mercury to the surface waters or where POTW sludge levels exceed or even approach regulatory limits, separators may serve a valid environmental purpose.

For dentists who want or need to install separators, as described above, we are providing our members the opportunity to learn more about separators at the Association's Annual Session in a couple of weeks. In addition, two articles about separators have been published in the monthly *Journal of the American Dental Association* (JADA), which is sent to all ADA members. In May 2002, the article titled "Laboratory Evaluation of Amalgam Separators" compared 12 separators that were on the market, showing that all 12 exceeded the International Organization for Standardization requirement of 95 percent amalgam removal efficiency. An article published in the August 2003 edition of *JADA*, titled "Purchasing, Installing and Operating Dental Amalgam Separators", provided dentists information on what to consider in choosing an amalgam separator as well as a more complete description of the short- and long-term costs of the available options.

Ultimately, we believe the most effective and responsible action we can take is to encourage state and local dental societies to work directly with the regulatory agencies that have responsibility for establishing local and state environmental policy. In this way, they can work together to find the most effective solution for their particular jurisdiction. If that solution includes the use of separators, we'll do our best to help our members comply.

National Advocacy Initiative

On April 18 of this year, the Association approached the Environmental Protection Agency (EPA) and proposed a "National Advocacy Initiative" with the goal of reducing amalgam waste releases into the environment. The action plan provides for the initiation of a dialogue with regulatory authorities so that a consensus on the appropriate approach of reducing dental amalgam discharges can be reached. The plan seeks to establish a national "guidance" for state and local regulators and dental societies, but expressly recognizes that more stringent requirements would apply where environmental conditions and regulatory requirements require more reductions.

Our plan includes the following:

<u>Recycling and the establishment of local bulk mercury collection programs</u>: We are proposing that EPA convene a working group consisting of the agency, ADA, interested state dental societies, state regulators, amalgam manufacturers and recyclers, and dental waste disposal companies to identify and eliminate barriers to recycling. In addition, the ADA supports local bulk collection programs, such as the Michigan program. The Association would be willing to discuss what, if any, role it can take to encourage such

activities. One of the possibilities is for the ADA and EPA to develop a model state or local recycling program.

Best Management Practices: The ADA will work with the EPA to implement the most effective ways to educate our members concerning the benefits of BMPs and encourage universal compliance.

ADA Education Program: The ADA would work with the EPA to develop a web page designed to educate dentists about environmental laws and to facilitate compliance. In addition to the web page, the ADA will educate dentists on reducing releases of amalgam from dental offices, legal requirements applicable to dentists, and other related matters via other means – these could include seminars, CDs, videos, printed brochures, articles in ADA publications and meetings with dental societies. In addition, we will work with the American Dental Education Association to develop model environmental protection curricula for dental schools.

National Dental Amalgam Minimization Plan: We are proposing that EPA work with the ADA to develop guidance that would recommend approaches for the states to take to encourage the reduction of amalgam discharges from dental offices to sewer systems. Once a final plan is issued, EPA will send it to the states and EPA regions. The ADA recognizes that under the provisions of the Clean Water Act states are allowed to be more stringent.

Inventory of Dental Amalgam and Releases: The ADA would compile information to prepare and maintain an inventory of dental amalgam use. The purpose is to track progress in reducing wastewater discharges of amalgam from dental offices. ADA would conduct member surveys to obtain information. EPA may also request information from amalgam manufacturers and recyclers.

Research: We suggest several areas where the EPA may want to provide support for further research.
- Develop joint ADA-EPA pilot projects for specific geographic locations (e.g. by state) to test the effectiveness of amalgam collection devices in capturing amalgam in dental offices prior to discharge.
- Research on more cost effective separator technology via a small business innovative technology research grant.
- Study the degree and mechanism by which amalgamated mercury may be methylated in a wastewater treatment plant and in the environment to become bioavailable.

Incentives to Participate in Voluntary Amalgam Reduction Programs: Working with EPA and state and local authorities, the ADA supports the establishment of incentives (e.g. grants to install mercury collection technology) for dentists to take voluntary amalgam reduction measures. The program would also provide individual dentists and state and local dental societies some concrete recognition of their efforts.

We are pleased to be able to report to the Subcommittee that the Association representatives have already begun a series of meetings with EPA officials to continue discussions about working together to implement elements of this initiative.

In closing, Mr. Chairman, thank you for this opportunity today to explain the actions the ADA is taking regarding amalgam waste discharges. I would be pleased to answer any questions at this time. Mr. Chairman, the ADA would also like to reserve the right to submit additional information for the record that we believe would be helpful to your inquiry.

ATTACHMENT 1

CONTRIBUTION OF HG FROM AIR DEPOSITION

WATERSHED	% FROM AIR DEPOSITION
Savannah River, GA	99% Savannah River, GA TMDL
Mermentau Basin, LA	99.4% EPA, TMDLs
Tacoma, Washington	99% EPA Mercury Advisory Committee Meeting
Vermilion-Teche Basin, LA	98.5% EPA TMDL
Great Lakes	97.5% to 91.3% (EPA, Regulatory Impact Analysis of the Final Great Lakes Water Quality Guidance)
Florida Everglades	95% USGS, *South Florida Science Forum*
Chesapeake Bay	50% 1998 EPA
Wisconsin Rivers	75% EPA Star Report
Calcasieu River Basin, LA	15.4% EPA TMDL for Calcasieu River Basin
Long Island	10% 1998 EPA

ATTACHEMENT 2:

COMPARISON OF HG RELEASES

SOURCE	EMISSION FROM DENTAL AMALGAM WASTE (EXCEPT WHERE NOTED)		
TOTAL HG RELEASED FROM AMALGAM WASTE	AIR EMITTED US (from incineration of sludge): 0.2 (ENVIRON) AIR DEPOSITED IN US: 0.1 (ENVIRON)[1] WATER: 0.3 (ENVIRON) TOTAL: **0.4** (ENVIRON) TOTAL BIOAVAILABLE = ? (assumed 100% bioavailable in ENVIRON)		
TOTAL US AIR EMISSIONS	EMITTED IN US. 158 (1995) 130 (2001)	DEPOSITED IN U.S. 53 (1995) 43 (2001)	Bioavailable ? ?

ATTACHMENT 3

MERCURY AIR EMISSIONS REDUCTION COSTS AND COST EFFECTIVENESS

SOURCE	TONS PER YEAR	COST-EFFECTIVENESS (MILLIONS OF DOLLARS PER TON)
AMALGAM WASTE SEPARATORS	~0.4	$273 to $1,700 (ENVIRON)
UTILITY **Coal**	~50	$134 to $140 (activated carbon) $70 (**Clear Skies,** based on DOE estimate of $24.4 billion cost for 70% reduction with a cost-effectiveness cap of $35,000 per pound) $1.6 billion per ton (Carper bill, based on DOE estimate of $65.4 billion cost for 79% reduction)
MUN. WASTE INCIN.	29.6	$0.411 TO $1.74
MED. WASTE INCIN.	16	$4 TO $8
CHLORO-ALKALI PLANTS	7.1	$9.18
REGULATION NOT COST-EFFECTIVE **CEMENT KILNS** **HAZARD. WASTE INCIN.**	4.4 7.1[14]	$20 to $50 $3.6 $9 (in rejecting beyond floor additional mercury controls)
EPA GREAT LAKES WATER QUALITY GUIDANCE (1995)	-	$2

Mr. BURTON. Mr. Berglund.

Mr. BERGLUND. Thank you, Mr. Chair.

My name is Peter Berglund. I'm with Metropolitan Council of POTW in St. Paul, MN, which in layman's terms I like to call it the sewer board.

We have completed two major research projects on dental clinics' loadings to sanitary sewers and the effectiveness of amalgam separators used to treat the clinic wastewater. The good news is that our loading estimates agree well with the ADA's ENVIRON report. We measured 234 milligrams of mercury per dentist per operating day and we also measured a 29 to 44 percent reduction in mercury loads at two of our treatment plants while amalgam separators were in place.

There is more good news. These reductions also agree well with the ADA's ENVIRON report. The ENVIRON report had showed dental contributions of approximately 50 percent to wastewater treatment plants. The bad news is that I had to handle this waste during my study.

We also studied and tested the separators in actual clinic settings. The ADA tested separators in a laboratory setting, so-called bench-top testing.

And there is more good news. Our results agree well with the ADA's testing of the separators. So both projects show that the separators perform well at removing amalgam from the wastewater.

Given all of this work which—I should mention our research projects were done in partnership with the Minnesota Dental Association. They helped us enormously on studying the loadings and studying the amalgam separators, so we continued that partnership on what we have called a voluntary dental office amalgam separator program to promote the installation of separators that remove 99 percent of the amalgam present in the wastewater. And we—in fact, we have—the results were so good in ADA's testing on the separators that we set the bar higher than the normal test criteria. We call for 99 percent removal of the amalgam in the wastewater where the common criteria is 95 percent.

We launched our program for the promotion of separator installation in January 2003, and we already have two-thirds of our dentists committed to installing separators. These are signed commitments sent in by the dentists. Two-thirds have sent that in. And many countries in the world call for separators, so this is not new.

I should mention that there've been reductions in mercury levels at wastewater treatment plants in, Toronto, Canada, and Wichita, KS, and the subcommittee may wish to get more information from those two cities.

Separators are effective at reducing the amount of amalgam discharged to treatment plants. The use of the separators in our area will drastically cut back the amount of mercury released via the burning of our sludge. And then for those treatment plants that may land apply, the sludge separators will obviously help reduce the amount of mercury present in that land-applied sludge. Capturing amalgam at a dental office will maximize the recycling of the mercury and the silver present in the amalgam. If these metals end up in a wastewater treatment plant sludge, they will not be recovered or reused.

One other little comment, the ADA environmental report had mentioned the possibility of dental clinic wastewater being discharged to septic tanks. We found in our early survey work that, yes, some dental waste does go into septic tanks, which is not allowed in Minnesota. The septic tank—septage from the septic tanks may be hauled back to the wastewater treatment plant, adding to the treatment plants' load, or it may be land applied. That concludes my comment.

Thank you.

Mr. BURTON. Thank you Mr. Berglund.

[The prepared statement of Mr. Berglund follows:]

October 8, 2003 Testimony before the
US Congress House Subcommittee on Human Rights and Wellness

Dental Mercury Loadings to Public Sewers,
Efficacy of Dental Amalgam Separators,
Metropolitan Council–Minnesota Dental Association Amalgam Separator Program

Metropolitan Council is the Publicly Owned Treatment Works for the Minneapolis/St. Paul, Minnesota metropolitan area, with the responsibility of treating wastewater. The Metropolitan Council (Council) has studied and identified sources of mercury discharged to the sanitary sewer since the mid 1990's.

Key Points:

(1) Dental offices are a significant contributor of mercury to sanitary sewers.
(2) Significant mercury reductions are anticipated at wastewater treatment plants if dental offices install amalgam separators.
(3) A joint program with the Council and the Minnesota Dental Association is underway to have dental offices install amalgam separators.

Dental offices are a source of mercury to the sanitary sewer due to the dental vacuum systems that collect and discharge amalgam wastes during dental office procedures. (Amalgam contains approximately one-half mercury; plus silver and other metals.) There are approximately 1361 general dentists in the Council's wastewater treatment plant service area. Data published in 1999 (WEF Monograph, co-authored by the Council) indicated that 4790 amalgam fillings are removed and 4870 new amalgam fillings are placed per work day in our service area. Using published data and Council survey findings the Council estimated a rate of mercury release of 255 mg/dentist/operating day, which indicated that approximately 75% of the mercury originated from dental offices (WEF 1999). Other sources were accounted for, thus completing a mass balance calculation.

Based on the initial estimated contribution from dental offices, the Council determined that it should conduct two studies to evaluate loadings from offices and to test "amalgam separators" designed to remove amalgam from office wastewater. To undertake these studies, the Council formed a partnership with the Minnesota Dental Association. Based on the two studies it was learned that the amount of mercury released from dental offices varies widely, with an average of 234 mg/dentist/operating day (Berglund and Diercks, 2001). It was also learned that the Council may be able to realize a 29% - 44% reduction in sludge mercury levels if dental offices install amalgam separators (Anderson, 2001). ("Sludge" refers to the solids generated during the treatment of wastewater.)

Using a four day workweek, and 48 weeks/year, the Council's preliminary calculation of data from the American Dental Association's ENVIRON report indicates a mercury release of 231 mg/dentist/operating day; based on 6.5 tons/year with 133,059 dentists (ENVIRON 2003). Therefore, the mercury loading values of 231–234–255 mg/dentist/operating day agree quite well.

The five amalgam separators that were tested by the Council and the Minnesota Dental Association in dental offices performed well and are cost-effective. There were no operational problems encountered during the test periods that separators were in the offices. The American Dental Association conducted bench-top testing in a laboratory setting, with results indicating that there are many separators that perform well. ADA's testing showed nine separators removing greater than 99% of the amalgam. Three other separators removed over 95% of the amalgam (Fan, et al., JADA 2002).

Therefore, the Council and the Minnesota Dental Association (MDA) have initiated a "Voluntary Dental Office Amalgam Separator Program" to promote the installation of separators that remove 99% of the amalgam present in dental office wastewater. (This is a higher percentage removal than called for in a standardized separator testing procedure.)

The Council-MDA program began in January 2003. Thanks to the efforts of the partnership with the MDA, two-thirds of the dental offices in the Minneapolis/St. Paul metropolitan area have already submitted signed commitments indicating that they will install a separator. MDA is also promoting this program throughout Minnesota, and they have achieved this same level of commitment statewide. Our goal is to have all general practice offices install a separator by February 2005. (Specialty dental offices are not expected to need a separator.)

Many countries in the world have programs that require the installation of amalgam separators, including Scandinavian countries, Germany, Switzerland, Austria, Holland, and Japan (as of approximately 1992). Many Danish sewer service areas have shown a reduction in sludge mercury levels. Approximately half of the service areas saw a reduction ranging from 14-80%. Apart from the one value of 14%, the range of the data was 32-80%. (The other half of the service areas observed no statistically significant changes.) (Arenholt-Bindslev, 1999)

Reductions in mercury levels at wastewater treatment plants have also been shown in Toronto and Wichita Kansas. The subcommittee may wish to contact these communities for more detailed information.

Separators are effective at reducing the amount of amalgam discharged to wastewater treatment plants. The use of separators will reduce the amount of mercury released to the atmosphere via the burning of sludge. For those treatment plants that land apply sludge, there will be less mercury present in the sludge, thereby maximizing the potential beneficial reuse of the sludge and the avoidance of costly alternative sludge disposal methods.

It should also be noted that most dental offices currently use one of two common types of vacuum systems. One type of system includes rudimentary, secondary filtration equipment. However, in some areas of the US, these types of vacuum systems are being phased out in favor of systems that use less water and electricity (so called, "dry" systems). Unfortunately, these "dry" vacuum systems usually do not filter out as much amalgam from the wastewater. If a dental office changes vacuum systems, it would be an ideal opportunity to install a separator. However, if the vacuum system is changed to a "dry" system, and a separator is not installed, there will be an increase in the amount of amalgam discharged to the sewer.

Capturing amalgam at a dental office will maximize recycling of mercury and silver present in amalgam. If these metals end up in wastewater treatment plant sludge, they will not be recovered or reused.

The ADA's ENVIRON report discusses dental office waste being discharged to septic tanks. The Council's survey work has also shown that some dental offices discharge to septic tanks (WEF 1999). Septic tank septage may be hauled to wastewater treatment plants adding to their load, or it may be land applied. Since some septic tanks overflow to a drainfield, this could be an environmental release from dental offices.

Testimony submitted by:
Peter Berglund, PE
Metropolitan Council Environmental Services (MCES, a division of the Metropolitan Council)
St. Paul, Minnesota   651-602-4708,   peter.berglund@metc.state.mn.us

References:

Anderson, C.T., (2001) Community-Wide Dental Mercury Study. *MCES and Minn. Dental Assoc. Report*, (MCES Report No. 01-507)

Arenholt-Bindslev, D. (1999) Environmental Aspects of Dental Restorative Materials: A Review of the Danish Situation. Proceedings of the AWMA, September 1999

Berglund, P.B. and Diercks, R.W. (2001), Evaluation of Amalgam Removal Equipment and Dental Clinic Loadings to the Sanitary Sewer. *MCES and Minn. Dental Assoc. Report*, (MCES Report No. 01-509)

ENVIRON International Corporation (2003), Assessment of Mercury in the Form of Amalgam in Dental Wastewater in the United States. (A report conducted at the request of the American Dental Association.)

Fan, P.L., et al. (2002) Laboratory Evaluation of Amalgam Separators. *The Journal of the American Dental Association* May 2002

WEF (1999) *Controlling Dental Facility Discharges in Wastewater*. Water Environment Federation, Alexandria VA

Mr. BURTON. Mr. LeBlanc.

Mr. LeBLANC. Good afternoon, Chairman Burton, members of the subcommittee. My name is Norm LeBlanc. I am chief of Technical Services for the Hampton Roads Sanitation District in Virginia Beach, VA, and Chair of the Association of Metropolitan Sewage Agencies [AMSA's], Water Quality Committee. AMSA represents the interests of nearly 300 of the Nation's wastewater treatment agencies, also known as publicly owned treatment works [POTWs].

AMSA members serve the majority of the sewer population of the United States, and I would like to thank you for the opportunity to present AMSA's position here at the subcommittee this afternoon.

Mr. Chairman, mercury is a multimedia problem that AMSA believes demands a multimedia, multifaceted solution. Only a coordinated effort involving all levels of government, Federal, State and local, will be able to address the mercury problem as a whole and be able to ensure that the resources being applied to control mercury across the Nation have a real impact on improving the environment and public health. AMSA, therefore, continues to support legislation that would create a national task force or some other type of interagency working group to evaluate the issues surrounding mercury in the environment and coordinating efforts to control it.

With that said, AMSA strongly believes that each wastewater treatment agency and the community they serve should have ultimate control over the approach used to reduce mercury discharges from dental offices. I hope my remarks today will provide you with added insight into what the Nation's POTWs are already doing to address the issue. The U.S. EPA's 1997 report to Congress on mercury demonstrated that when compared to all of the sources of mercury released to the environment, wastewater treatment facilities are de minimis sources, or minor sources. Despite their de minimis contributions, wastewater treatment agencies continue to receive stringent numeric limits for mercury in their wastewater discharge permits, and many are experiencing difficulties in complying with these new limits.

I want to be clear that POTWs want to do their part in reducing mercury releases to the environment, but it is important to recognize that wastewater treatment plants are not designed to remove toxics like mercury. In fact, the Clean Water Act, in requiring us to implement pretreatment programs, recognizes that it's not only good public policy, but also good engineering practice to remove toxins at the source and not at the wastewater treatment plant.

A well-run pretreatment program is a POTW's first and, primarily, its only line of defense against toxic discharges; and it's critical for reducing mercury concentrations in wastewater discharge to the environment. Although residential sources of mercury, such as human waste and household products, are significant, POTWs have absolutely no authority to control these sources.

Dental office mercury, which makes up about 40 percent of the mercury coming into the wastewater treatment plant, according to a March 2002 AMSA study and a recent ADA report, is controllable. Consequently, dental offices will almost always be a component of pretreatment efforts to control mercury in order to meet permit limits.

Pretreatment programs can approach the issue of dental office mercury control in many ways, and AMSA believes that each community will choose the approach that works best for it. While some communities may have chosen the approach of issuing voluntary best-management practices that dental offices are asked to implement, other communities are requiring dental offices to install equipment such as amalgam separators to remove the mercury contained in amalgam fillings before it has a chance to enter the sewer system.

There are success stories for each type of approach where reductions have been made in the amount of mercury being discharged to the wastewater treatment plant. In most communities, it's too early to tell whether or not long-term implementation of these programs will achieve the low levels of mercury necessary to meet increasingly stringent permit limits, but preliminary indications are that they will not.

More work is needed to evaluate the options available for controlling the amount of mercury entering POTWs, and AMSA has recently begun a new international study to evaluate the effectiveness of amalgam separators at reducing mercury load from dental offices. This project, however, will not be completed until 2005.

AMSA's 2002 study on the effectiveness of pollution prevention in our source control by reducing mercury discharged to wastewater treatment plants does suggest that pollution prevention efforts alone, without the use of amalgam separators, for example, will not enable POTWs to meet stringent permit limits.

AMSA had recently had the opportunity to peer review the ADA assessment on the quantity of mercury nationwide that finds its way into the environment from dental offices. While a review on the final report is still ongoing, many of AMSA's were addressed in the final document, nevertheless some broader issues remain that we feel the report could have addressed better, and AMSA will be providing additional comments to the ADA on those issues.

The Nation's wastewater treatment agencies continue to do their best to minimize the discharge of mercury to their plants and, subsequently, to the environment from all potential controllable sources, including dental offices. It is important that we have the ability to control all commercial industrial sources of mercury if we are to have any chance of meeting current and future requirements. However, we do not want to mislead the subcommittee into believing that controlling dental offices alone will result in attainment of Clean Water Act requirements at all POTWs.

AMSA looks forward to working with you and your colleagues, as well as the national and State dental associations on mercury issues, and appreciates the opportunity to provide our expertise on mercury to the subcommittee. And I'll be happy to answer any questions.

Mr. BURTON. Thank you.

[The prepared statement of Mr. LeBlanc follows:]

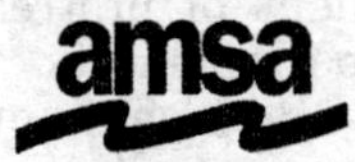

Association of
Metropolitan
Sewerage Agencies

TESTIMONY OF THE

ASSOCIATION OF METROPOLITAN SEWERAGE AGENCIES
(AMSA)

October 8, 2003

Presented by

Norman LeBlanc
Chief, Technical Services

Hampton Roads Sanitation District
Virginia Beach, Virginia

Submitted to
the
SUBCOMMITTEE ON HUMAN RIGHTS AND WELLNESS

COMMITTEE ON GOVERNMENT REFORM

WASHINGTON, DC

1816 Jefferson Place, NW
Washington, DC 20036-2505
202.833.AMSA
202.833.4657 FAX
info@amsa-cleanwater.org

Testimony of Norman LeBlanc
Chief, Technical Services, Hampton Roads Sanitation District
on behalf of the
Association of Metropolitan Sewerage Agencies

Good afternoon Chairman Burton, Congresswoman Watson and members of the Subcommittee, my name is Norm LeBlanc. I am Chief of Technical Services for the Hampton Roads Sanitation District, in Virginia Beach, Virginia and Chair of the Association of Metropolitan Sewerage Agencies' (AMSA) Water Quality Committee. Founded in 1970, AMSA represents the interests of nearly 300 of the nation's wastewater treatment agencies, also known as publicly owned treatment works or POTWs. AMSA members serve the majority of the sewered population in the United States and collectively treat and reclaim over 18 billion gallons of wastewater every day.

Thank you for the opportunity to present AMSA's perspective on this very important issue. AMSA is actively engaged in the national dialogue on mercury. Through the efforts of its Mercury Workgroup, AMSA continues to explore effective and reasonable approaches to controlling mercury discharges to the nation's waters.

Mercury is an important issue that publicly owned treatment works have been tracking for over 20 years. The largest sources of mercury to the environment are air deposition from coal-fired utilities in the east and legacy mining wastes in the west. In its December 1997 *Mercury Study Report to Congress*, the U.S. Environmental Protection Agency (EPA) demonstrated that when compared to all other sources of mercury released to the environment, wastewater treatment facilities are a minor or *de minimis* source. Yet the regulatory focus has been on entities like POTWs that receive permits from the states or EPA to discharge to the nation's waters. The largest sources of mercury in the environment are, for the most part, unregulated.

Despite their *de minimis* contribution, over the past several years, more and more wastewater treatment agencies have begun to receive stringent numeric limits for mercury in wastewater discharge permits issued by the states or EPA. Because we have new, very sensitive analytical methods for detecting mercury in wastewater, many of these wastewater treatment agencies are experiencing difficulties in complying with the new limits, which are at the part per trillion level (a part per trillion is equivalent to a grain of sand in an Olympic-sized swimming pool). Studies conducted in Ohio and California have shown that even if POTWs install sophisticated, costly treatment similar to desalination technologies, in other words spend billions of dollars to remove a few pounds of mercury, it will not be possible to meet these stringent limits, and the treatment residue would be hazardous and difficult to manage.

I want to be clear that POTWs want to do their part in reducing mercury releases to the environment. But, it is important to recognize that wastewater treatment plants are not designed to remove toxics like mercury. In fact, the Clean Water Act recognizes that toxics are not to be removed by POTWs and mandates that the nation's wastewater treatment agencies implement pretreatment programs to remove toxic constituents before they enter the treatment plant. Pretreatment programs recognize that it is more efficient to remove toxics at their sources rather than wait until they are diluted into millions of gallons of wastewater. Pretreatment programs seek out the toxics at their sources and place limits on the discharge of those toxics into the sewer system. A well-run pretreatment program is a POTW's first and, sometimes, only line of defense against toxic discharges and is critical for reducing mercury concentrations in wastewater discharged to the environment. In the case of mercury, most pretreatment programs ultimately recognize the need to address dental office discharges.

AMSA's Mercury Workgroup was formed to ensure that AMSA members have access to the latest information on mercury issues and to provide a venue for sharing expertise and experience. Where information has not been readily available, AMSA's Mercury Workgroup has conducted its own studies and generated its own reports to provide its members with the information they need to address mercury.

A March 2002 AMSA study entitled, *Mercury Source Control and Pollution Prevention Program Evaluation,* conducted under a cooperative agreement with EPA, found that on average, 35-40% of the mercury coming into a POTW's treatment plant is attributable to dental offices. While human waste and food products are significant sources of mercury, they are not controllable. Consequently, dental offices must be a component of most pretreatment efforts to control mercury. Pretreatment programs can approach the issue of dental office mercury control in many different ways, and AMSA believes that each community will choose the approach that works best for it. While some communities have chosen to approach the issue using voluntary, best management practices that dental offices are asked to implement, other communities are requiring dental offices to install equipment, such as amalgam separators, to remove the mercury contained in amalgam (e.g., silver) fillings before it enters the sewer system.

AMSA's March 2002 report on the effectiveness of traditional source control and pollution prevention efforts in decreasing the mercury discharges to POTWs concluded that while these efforts may significantly decrease the amount of mercury entering a wastewater treatment plant, pollution prevention and source control alone will not enable wastewater treatment agencies to meet extremely low mercury limits. More work is needed to evaluate the options available for controlling the amount of mercury entering POTWs and AMSA has recently begun a new, international study to evaluate the effectiveness of amalgam separators at reducing the mercury load from dental offices. This work will not be completed until the middle of 2005, but AMSA is certain that the results of the study will help to inform communities as they decide what approach is right for them.

AMSA recently had the opportunity to peer review an American Dental Association (ADA) assessment of the quantity of mercury nationwide that finds its way into the environment from dental offices. AMSA appreciated the ADA's invitation to review and comment on the report and assembled a team of wastewater treatment experts to review the document. While our review of the final report is still ongoing, I can tell you that many of AMSA's comments on the draft report were addressed in the final document. One of AMSA's primary concerns with the initial draft of the report was the lack of acknowledgement that dental offices are a major source of mercury for POTWs. AMSA was pleased to see that in the final report, the ADA acknowledged that approximately 40-50% of the mercury received by POTWs comes from dentists. Nevertheless, some broader issues remain that we feel the final report could have addressed better, specifically the ADA's claim that dental amalgam separators are not needed in dental offices because the mercury captured by the separators would be the same mercury that is incidentally removed during wastewater treatment. AMSA's new study on amalgam separator effectiveness should shed some light on this issue.

AMSA and its members continue to do their best to minimize the discharge of mercury to POTWs from all sources, including dental offices. AMSA's Mercury Workgroup continues to develop resources and conduct studies to provide further insight into the mercury issue including the studies I mentioned previously and several other efforts, most notably our August 2000 report, *Evaluation of Domestic Sources of Mercury*, which highlighted that mercury from residential sources, including many household products and human wastes, can be a significant source of mercury to POTWs.

While AMSA strongly believes that, as necessary, each wastewater treatment agency should develop a program for controlling mercury from dental offices that meets the needs of its community, and that a single, national approach to controlling dental office mercury discharges will not provide the flexibility necessary to address the characteristics of each community, AMSA also understands that the mercury issue extends well beyond dental offices.

Mr. Chairman, mercury is a multi-media problem that AMSA believes demands a multi-media, multi-faceted solution. Only a national strategy for addressing the mercury problem as a whole, whether it is air deposition, mining wastes, federal stockpiles, or discharges to the nation's waters, will be able to ensure that the resources being applied to control mercury across the nation have a real impact on improving the environment and protecting public health. AMSA, therefore, continues to support legislation that would create a national task force or some other type of inter-agency working group to evaluate the issues surrounding mercury in the environment.

AMSA looks forward to working with you and your colleagues as well as the national and state dental associations on mercury issues and appreciates the opportunity to provide our expertise on mercury to the Subcommittee. At this time, I will be happy to answer any questions.

Mr. BURTON. Mr. Galvin.

Mr. GALVIN. Chairman Burton, my name is David Galvin. I'm a program manager with King County's Department of Natural Resources and Parks based in Seattle, WA.

King County operates the major wastewater treatment system for the Metro Seattle area, including two large treatment plants with total flows of about 200 million gallons per day. We discharge treated effluent into Puget Sound, a sensitive marine waterway.

One hundred percent of the residual solids from our treatment plants, known as biosolids, is reused beneficially in wheat and hop fields in eastern Washington and forestlands in the Cascade Mountains and in the composted product available for landscaping. We control sources of contaminants into our system by means of a major industrial pretreatment program and extensive work with small businesses and households.

Toxic metals, including mercury, don't go away or get magically treated in wastewater treatment plants. Rather, they either settle out in the solids or are discharged in the water effluent. Most mercury that enters our system ends up in our biosolids. Even though our biosolids currently meet Federal and State regulations for mercury, our concerns for the future marketability of these solids drives our efforts to continuously make them cleaner. But potential for more stringent mercury limits in the future is also a concern for us.

Under an agreement with the Seattle-King County Dental Society, we conducted an extensive collaborative program from 1995 through 2000 to promote voluntary compliance of the dental offices in our area. We encouraged purchasing an installation of amalgam separator units, which research showed would allow dentists to meet King County's local mercury limit. The results after 6 years of this collaborative voluntary approach were that 24 dental offices, out of approximately 900, installed amalgam separators.

In 2001, King County in consultation with the local dental society decided that the voluntary program had failed and notified local dentists that they would be required to meet our local discharge limit. We gave them the choice of installing separators or applying for a permit and proving that they can meet our limits without a separator.

We gave them 2 years to meet compliance, until July 1, 2003. We provided extensive outreach to these dental offices, including technical assistance, via visits from our public health staff to every dental office in the county. We provided monetary incentives via vouchers reimbursed at 50 percent of the costs up to $500. We worked closely with the local dental society as they held trade fairs and technical workshops.

Local dentists did not fight this new requirement, but rather, sought practical information about purchasing separators, and they got on with the task. Results in the 2 years since the requirement was announced are that approximately 750 additional dental offices, that is, more than 80 percent, have installed amalgam separator units, with the remaining offices quickly following suit during this last quarter.

In conclusion, we believe that mercury is best controlled at the dental office, not at the wastewater treatment plant. Control at the source is the best way to manage such toxic metals. A voluntary program did not result in significant change in King County. Once separators were mandated, compliance happened quickly, dramatically and with little resistance.

Amalgam separator units are effective at removing at least 95 percent of the mercury. They are readily available, low tech, reasonably priced and easily installed and maintained.

The attached graph that I included with my testimony shows the results of our work, both in the voluntary phase and once we made it a requirement.

Thank you for the opportunity to testify. I would be happy to answer any questions.

Mr. BURTON. Thank you, Mr. Galvin.

[The prepared statement of Mr. Galvin follows:]

King County
Department of Natural Resources and Parks
Water and Land Resources Division
Hazardous Waste Management Program
130 Nickerson Street, Suite 100
Seattle, WA 98109-1658
206-263-3050

Testimony of David V. Galvin, King County, Washington, to the U.S. House of Representatives, Subcommittee on Human Rights and Wellness of the Committee on Government Reform, at its hearing on "The Environmental Impact of Mercury-Containing Dental Amalgam," held October 8, 2003.

My name is David Galvin and I am a program manager for King County's Department of Natural Resources and Parks, based in Seattle, Washington. King County operates the major wastewater treatment system for the metropolitan Seattle area, including two large wastewater treatment plants with total average flows of 200 million gallons per day. We discharge treated effluent into Puget Sound, a sensitive marine waterway. One-hundred percent of the residual solids from our treatment plants, known as biosolids, is reused beneficially in wheat and hop fields in Eastern Washington, on forest lands in the Cascade Mountains, and in a composted product available for landscaping. We control sources of contaminants into our system, by means of a major industrial pretreatment program and extensive work with small businesses and households.

Toxic metals, including mercury, don't go away or get magically "treated" in wastewater treatment plants; rather, they either settle out into the solids or are discharged in the water effluent. Most mercury that enters our system ends up in the biosolids. Even though our biosolids currently meet all federal and state regulations for mercury, our concerns for future marketability of these solids drives our efforts to continuously make them cleaner. The potential for more stringent mercury limits in the future is also of concern.

Under an agreement with the Seattle-King County Dental Society, we conducted an extensive, collaborative program from 1995 through 2000 to promote voluntary compliance. We encouraged purchase and installation of amalgam separator units, which research showed would allow dentists to meet King County's local mercury limit. The results after six years were that 24 dental offices, out of approximately 900, installed amalgam separators.

In 2001, King County in consultation with the local dental society decided that the voluntary program had failed and notified local dentists that they would be required to meet our local discharge limit of 0.2 parts per million total mercury. We gave them the choice of installing separators or applying for a permit and proving they meet our limits without a separator. We gave them two years to meet compliance – until July 1, 2003.

We provided extensive outreach to the dental offices, including technical assistance site visits by staff from Public Health - Seattle & King County to every office in the county. We provided monetary incentives via vouchers reimbursed at 50% of costs up to $500. We worked closely with the local dental society as they held trade fairs and technical workshops. Local dentists did not fight this requirement, but rather sought practical information about purchasing separators and got on with the task. Results in the two years since the requirement was announced: approximately 750 additional dental offices (more than 80%) installed amalgam separator units, with the remaining offices quickly following suit in this last quarter.

In conclusion:
- Mercury is best controlled at the dental office, not at the wastewater treatment plant. Control at the source is the best way to manage such toxic metals.
- A voluntary program did not result in significant change in King County. Once separators were mandated, compliance happened quickly, dramatically and with little resistance.
- Amalgam separator units are effective at removing 95% of mercury; they are readily available, low tech, reasonably priced and easily installed and maintained.
- The attached graph illustrates our experience.

Thank you for the opportunity to testify today. I would be happy to answer any questions from the committee members.

King County
Department of Natural Resources and Parks
Water and Land Resources Division
Hazardous Waste Management Program
130 Nickerson Street, Suite 100
Seattle, WA 98109-1658
206-263-3050

Managing Wastewater from Dental Offices
King County, Washington's Experience

Background for testimony presented by David Galvin, King County Department of Natural Resources and Parks, Seattle, Washington at the hearing on "The Environmental Impact of Mercury-Containing Dental Amalgam," U.S. House of Representatives Subcommittee on Human Rights and Wellness of the Committee on Government Reform, October 8, 2003.

King County's Wastewater Treatment System: An Overview

King County operates a regional wastewater collection and treatment system with two major treatment plants. The 420-square mile service area includes metropolitan Seattle, most of urbanized King County and parts of south Snohomish County. The wastewater treatment system, with an average flow of 200 million gallons per day, serves approximately 1.4 million people. Ninety-five percent of the flow comes from residential homes and small businesses and five percent from industrial sources. The treatment system serves an estimated 1400 general practice dentists in 900 general practice dental offices.

King County's wastewater treatment system discharges treated effluent into Puget Sound, a sensitive marine waterway. Residual solids from the two treatment plants, known as biosolids, are land-applied on wheat and hop fields in Eastern Washington and on forestlands in the Cascade Mountains. Some are sold as a composted product available for landscaping.

Wastewater treatment plants aren't designed to handle toxic metals, like mercury. Heavy metals that enter the treatment system don't go away, or get magically 'treated.' Rather, they collect in the sewer lines, settle out in the solids, or are discharged in the water effluent (to Puget Sound). Most mercury entering King County's treatment system ends up in the biosolids. King County actively controls contaminants, including mercury, entering the wastewater system by means of a major industrial pretreatment program and extensive work with small businesses and households.

While King County's biosolids currently meet all federal and state limits for mercury, an ongoing need to protect the future marketability of these solids drives the County's efforts to continuously make them cleaner. In addition, the possibility of more stringent mercury effluent limits—such as those imposed in the Great Lakes region—motivates King County's efforts to remove this contaminant at the source.

1991 – 2000: Attempts to Manage Mercury Discharges from Dental Offices

Attention turned to dentists in the early 1990's, when the Washington State Department of Ecology noted occasional high levels of mercury in the King County wastewater treatment system and required Metro, the wastewater treatment agency (now King County), to reduce discharges of mercury at the source. Because of their numbers, dentists were considered a potentially significant source of mercury, and a 1991 study confirmed that the dental sector was indeed a "significant and identifiable" source of mercury to the wastewater system.[1] (These findings have subsequently been corroborated in other municipalities.[2])

Source control in a dental office means settling or otherwise capturing mercury-bearing amalgam particles from wastewater before discharge to the sewer system. In the early 1990's, only a few amalgam separation units—manufactured in Europe—were available. During the period 1991-94, Metro (now King County) reviewed available separation units for their effectiveness, developed a set of considerations by which to evaluate separation units, and published a hazardous waste guidebook for dentists.

1994: Proposed 'Rule' Mandating Amalgam Separators. In early 1994 Metro/King County proposed a rule requiring dental offices to install amalgam separation equipment to demonstrate compliance with local discharge limits for mercury (that is, 0.2 milligrams per liter [mg/L], or 0.2 parts per million.) Due to a number of factors, including information received during the public comment period and pressure from organized dentistry, Metro/King County decided to forego the rule. Instead, the agency agreed to work cooperatively with the dental community to achieve voluntary compliance.

> ". . . the King County Department of Metropolitan Services (Metro) has decided to postpone promulgating the rule. Rather than establish the mechanisms required for regulatory compliance, Metro will promote voluntary compliance by continuing to work cooperatively with the dental community.
>
> Many dental offices have already installed amalgam separation units and we expect this practice to continue without a formal regulatory requirement. We believe this decision is in our community's best interest because it is cost effective and protects our environment. If information contradicts this decision in the future, we will reconsider promulgation of a rule at that time."[3]

---

[1] Metro (1991). (Municipality of Metropolitan Seattle) (now King County). Reported titled Dental Office Waste Stream Characterization Study. Contact Cynthia Balogh at 206-263-3075. Cynthia.balogh@mctrokc.gov .

[2] Chapman, P. and McGroddy, S. (nd) Report titled "Bioavailability of mercury from dental amalgam." Contact: Capital Regional District, 524 Yates St., PO Box 1000, Victoria, British Columbia V8W 2S6 Canada..

[3] Grigsby, D. (1995) Director, Water Pollution Control Department, Municipality of Metropolitan Seattle. Memo dated February 3, 1995.

One reason for postponing the rule was that amalgam separators developed in Europe were not readily available on the West Coast. Given more time, it was assumed that separators would become more available: they would be cheaper, more effective, better serviced and more reliable. In addition, dentists expressed interest in voluntarily controlling their mercury discharges—*if given time to do this*. The local dental society expressed a willingness to collaborate on the issue.

1995 – 2000: Outreach, Education and Voluntary Compliance. In collaboration with the local dental society, King County conducted an extensive outreach program to promote voluntary compliance in the management of amalgam wastes and wastewater during the period 1995 - 2000. Specifically, the Seattle-King County Dental Society and the King County Hazardous Waste Management Program worked on a variety of fronts to educate dentists about the need to properly manage amalgam wastes and to install separators. Activities during the six-year period include:
- Articles and paid advertisements in the Seattle-King County Dental Society *Journal*;
- *Handling Dental Wastes Poster* (7 editions), mailed to all members of the Society;
- *Dental Waste Management Guidebook,* developed, published and provided to all dental offices;
- Presentations/workshops at dental conventions, study groups and Society meetings;
- Cash rebates (subsidized by the County) for purchase of amalgam separators;
- Newspaper articles acknowledging 'green' dentists;
- Outreach to dental supply companies;
- Curriculum prepared for dental assistant/hygienist training programs;
- Technical assistance visits to dental offices.

Of special note, the County, the dental society, and three hazardous waste service providers collaborated to provide a one-time *free* waste pick up for dental offices in 1999. The County underwrote pick up and disposal costs, the Society promoted the project and screened applicants, and the waste haulers offered a special rate. An ongoing County voucher incentive program provided matching funds (in the form of rebates) to dental offices that purchased amalgam separators and/or contracted with waste management service providers.

As a result of these efforts, the Seattle-King County Dental Society won a "Golden Apple" award from a professional association and a Waste Information Network Environmental Achievement Award.

2000: Evaluation of the Voluntary Program. In 1999-2000, 212 dental offices in several representative zip code areas in King County received visits by King County staff to assess disposal practices for amalgam and other wastes. In addition, manufacturers of amalgam separation equipment provided sales data about installations of separators. These data provide a basis to evaluate whether the voluntary compliance program was effective. Results are summarized in a King County report.[4]

Briefly, the study showed that less than half of King County dentists collected and properly disposed of their waste amalgam solids—38 percent properly handled scrap amalgam, 27 percent properly handled amalgam from chairside traps, and only 13 percent properly handled amalgam in pump filters.

---

[4] Local Hazardous Waste Management Program in King County, 2000. "Management of hazardous dental wastes in King County, 1991-2000." King County Dept. of Natural Resources, Seattle, WA.

More significantly, only 24 of an estimated 900 dental offices had installed amalgam separators—that is, less than 3 percent of offices needing separators had installed them.

In 2001, King County, in consultation with the Seattle-King County Dental Society, concluded that the voluntary program had failed. King County then notified dentists that they would be required to meet local discharge limits of 0.2 parts per million total mercury.

2001 – 2003: King County Dentists Required to Meet Discharge Limits

Because the voluntary program failed to achieve compliance in managing dental wastewater—less than three percent of dental offices had installed separators—King County established a mandatory compliance schedule for dental offices in June 2001. This schedule required dental offices to comply with local discharge limits for mercury by July 1, 2003.

The decision to regulate dental offices was made because King County, as a delegated pretreatment program, is required to enforce regulations mandated under state and federal laws. Additionally, the marketability of biosolids is of critical importance to King County (a mandated goal is "to improve opportunities for recycling and reclamation of wastewater and biosolids" [K.C. Code 28.81.020]). King County land-applies approximately 130,000 wet tons of biosolids each year at a cost of $32 per wet ton. If biosolids weren't land-applied, the cost to landfill them would rise to $90 per wet ton. Public perception and future regulatory uncertainty make it imperative that King County use its resources to continually improve the biosolids quality.

In July 2001, King County informed dental offices served by the King County treatment system that they must comply with local discharge limits for mercury (0.2 mg/L or 0.2 ppm). Letters and fact sheets with instructions on how to meet the limits were sent to all dentists. In addition, the Seattle-King County Dental Society inserted a copy of the fact sheet in their July newsletter.

From August 2001 to July 2003, inspectors from Public Health – Seattle & King County, working as part of the Local Hazardous Waste Management Program, visited King County dental offices to explain the regulations and to assist dentists in getting their practices into compliance. In fall 2003, inspections to determine the compliance status of dental offices will begin; a portion of dental practices will be inspected each year thereafter.

Compliance Requirements. In King County, a dental office can demonstrate compliance with sewer limits if it: a) follows Best Management Practices for amalgam wastes (these are detailed in the fact sheet); b) properly handles used X-ray fixer; and c) installs amalgam separation equipment approved by King County *or* obtains a permit to discharge in King County. (In most cases, dental offices that apply for a permit must sample their wastewater to demonstrate that it meets the local limit for mercury.) Fact sheets, permit applications and other documents are available on the King County Web site.[5]

Exempt Specialties: King County specifically exempts certain specialties from the requirement of installing an amalgam separator or obtaining a permit. These are periodontics, orthodontics, oral

---

[5] See King County Web site at http://dnr.metrokc.gov/wlr/indwaste/dentists.htm

pathology/oral medicine, oral and maxillofacial surgery, radiology, and prosthodontists and endodontists that do not place and remove amalgam as a courtesy for their clients. Dentists that place or remove amalgam on three days or less each year are also exempt. (This latter exemption most often applies to pediatric dentists that don't place amalgams.) While dental offices that fall under the exemption don't need to install a separator or apply for a permit, they must follow best management practices, and they may be inspected.

Assistance to Dentists: Compliance assistance was provided to the King County dental community in a number of ways. As noted above, inspectors from Public Health – Seattle & King County, working as part of the Local Hazardous Waste Management Program, visited every dental office to explain the regulations and provide other technical assistance. This face-to-face contact appeared to be helpful in promoting proper management of a number of wastes of interest to King County in addition to amalgam wastewater (e.g., X-ray fixer containing silver, amalgam scrap, lead foils and instrument sterilants.)

The Voucher Incentive Program—essentially a matching fund rebate program subsidized by the County—was used to promote the purchase of amalgam separators during the first year of the program (it was discontinued in 2003). Approximately 371 vouchers (totaling $162,000) were redeemed by dentists to buy amalgam separators.

King County maintained a Web site explaining the regulations and compliance requirements.[6] Amalgam separators approved by the County were listed on the site, and a list of hazardous waste management firms was provided. A permit application could be downloaded from the site.

The Seattle-King County Dental Association provided regular information about requirements in its monthly newsletter and held two dinner meetings at which separator manufacturers introduced their products. The manufacturers of amalgam separation equipment marketed their products through advertisements, direct mail and dental supply firms.

Results of Mandatory Program: The deadline for dental offices to achieve compliance with King County's local limit for mercury was June 30, 2003. To monitor compliance, King County will perform random compliance inspections with a budget of $55,000 the first year. The County's goal is to maintain the program with existing staff and at a minimal cost by inspecting a certain percentage of businesses each year, handling these inspections in conjunction with other field work.

Aggregate sales data from manufacturers of amalgam separators indicate that more than 775 dental offices had installed amalgam separators as of June 30, 2003. (This is more than 85 percent of the 900 dental offices estimated to need separators to meet mercury discharge limits.) Purchases of amalgam separators by dental offices rose dramatically after the July 2001 letter requiring compliance with discharge limits was sent (see Table 1).

There was little—if any—resistance from the dental community about compliance requirements. The Seattle-King County Dental Society assumed a role of providing information to member dentists via its newsletter and meetings. The Washington State Dental Association requested clarification about particular legal requirements. Individual dentists, for the most part, were interested in the practical issues of how, where and what type of separators to buy.

---

[6] See King County Web site at http://dnr.metrokc.gov/wlr/indwaste/dentists.htm

As of the compliance date, King County had received fewer than 20 applications for permits from dental practices that didn't need to install separators. One dentist was issued a permit and the rest will be issued letters of exemption, as they did not readily fit into any category.

Table 1 Dental Offices Installing Separators in King County

1994 – 1999	24
2000	2
Jan – June 2001	5
July – Dec 2001	53*
Jan – June 2002	150
July – Dec 2002	286
Jan – June 2003	259

* Letter mailed in July 200**

Sources

Chapman, P. and McGroddy, S. (nd) Report titled "Bioavailability of mercury from dental amalgam." Contact: Capital Regional District, 524 Yates St., PO Box 1000, Victoria, British Columbia V8W 2S6 Canada.

Grigsby, D. (1995) Director, Water Pollution Control Department, Municipality of Metropolitan Seattle. Memo dated February 3, 1995.

Metro (1991). (Municipality of Metropolitan Seattle) (now King County). Reported titled Dental Office Waste Stream Characterization Study. Contact Cynthia Balogh at 206-263-3075. Cynthia.balogh@metrokc.gov .

Local Hazardous Waste Management Program in King County, 2000. "Management of hazardous dental wastes in King County, 1991-2000." King County Dept. of Natural Resources, Seattle, WA.

Mr. BURTON. Dr. Eichmiller, you read that resolution that you hope will be adopted at the ADA meeting, and it was voluntary. Did you just get those figures that he cited from the State of Washington?

Dr. EICHMILLER. Yes, I did.

Mr. BURTON. Twenty-four out of 900-some dentists complied after 6 years?

Dr. EICHMILLER. That's correct, sir.

Mr. BURTON. What makes you think that a voluntary resolution is going to bear fruit?

Dr. EICHMILLER. Well, I should also say that where separators are mandated, such as this, we have—and I think it was a good example—we have worked directly with the regulator to try to disseminate the information and to try to implement that. So we definitely want to facilitate the use of those separators when they are mandated on that local level.

What we're opposing is a mandate on a national scale.

Mr. BURTON. Why?

Dr. EICHMILLER. One is that there really is—and I think from the EPA's testimony, too, they pointed out that there wasn't a one-size-fits-all. The regulatory process here is one that is done on a local and regional level, and what we found to be most effective is when we work with those local and regional regulators to come up with programs that perhaps will include separators, but also include all the best management practices and all the education and outreach that have to go with it. And that, I think, attests to the success they had in the second round. We have also seen that in other areas where we have used this approach.

Mr. BURTON. Mr. LeBlanc, you said that the safety approaches that are being used by dentists, I guess on a voluntary basis now, have not or you don't believe will appreciably change the amount of mercury that is going into the wastewater treatment plants.

Mr. LEBLANC. I'm sorry. I think you misunderstood what I said.

Mr. BURTON. Well, you said 40 percent of the——

Mr. LEBLANC. I said dentists contributed about 40 percent of the total load of mercury to the POTWs. There are success stories, I think, out there that deal with voluntary programs; and there are stories, there are areas where mandatory requirements are necessary.

The need to control mercury and to what level it needs to be controlled is somewhat a function of the discharge situation, the area of the country, the relative sources of where you are in terms of meeting your regulatory requirements.

Mr. BURTON. But you continued to have substantial amounts of mercury in the wastewater treatments plants in your area?

Mr. LEBLANC. We have a voluntary program; we have seen reductions in our area, in the Hampton Roads Sanitation District area. And we do not mandate it as a requirement. We currently meet all of our, exceed all of our regulatory—"exceed" is a bad word; we better our requirements, our regulatory requirements, without mandating amalgam separators with the exception of the naval facility that you talked about earlier.

Mr. BURTON. The problem that they had down there with the inordinate amount of mercury coming into the sewage treatment plant from that facility down there, that dental facility where you had to put them in 90-gallon drums and haul them away, you don't have that problem any longer?

Mr. LeBlanc. Yes, we do.

Mr. Burton. Oh, you do? Why?

Mr. LeBlanc. Well, first of all, let me put that in perspective a little bit.

That is a unique situation where we have a relatively small treatment facility that is designed to treat a population of about 100,000 people, 18 million gallons a day. And it handles the naval operations base, Norfolk, the world's largest naval facility which houses, I understand, if not the largest, one of the largest dental clinics in the United States. It has the equivalent of 100 dentists' offices in—for a city the size of 100,000 people, which is a lot of dentists for a fairly small area.

A local limit was established at that plant to protect the biosolids for land application. Even though we incinerate that—biosolids at that plant, our policy at Hampton Roads Sanitation District is to have quality of our biosolids sufficient to allow us to use all options to handle our biosolids. So we set a fairly stringent limit to get the mercury in the biosolids at that plant down.

The Navy had a great deal of difficulty meeting that local limit. And while it's improved and they've tried numerous technologies over the years and have gotten better, they still cannot consistently meet the limit for that facility because it is fairly—it is very stringent. It's probably one of the most stringent in the Nation. And they are currently still barreling it up right now.

Mr. Burton. Mr. Galvin, based upon your experience in the State of Washington, do you think that any part of the country would have better results on a voluntary program of having dentists comply?

Mr. Galvin. I haven't had experience working with dentists from other parts of the country. The dentists that we've worked with in the Seattle-King County area are professionals, and they've been fine to work with. Our experience has been, even after years of a very collaborative process working with their dental society and a lot of site visits, that proof of the actual number of separators installed was still only about—less than 3 percent of the total number of dental offices in our system. And once we said that isn't working, we need to make this a requirement, then the compliance has been very good.

Mr. Burton. Well, if we didn't have mercury amalgams in our teeth, you wouldn't have that problem with having to haul away, in 98 gallon drums, that sludge, would you?

Mr. Galvin. You're correct.

Mr. Burton. So the mercury amalgams in those people's teeth that are being put in the trash and the sewage treatment plant is a problem. And if it wasn't there, it wouldn't be a problem. And the thing that everybody keeps defending is that in our mouths it's safe.

You know, I was always taught that if you're going to err, you err on the side of caution. You don't continue to say, well, you know, there's only a 5 percent chance that you're going to die from this, or a 10 percent chance. If there's a possibility of making it 100 percent safe, why would you keep people in the situation where there's a 10 percent or 20 percent or 5 percent chance of having neurological problems from the substance that you're putting into their bodies.

We see mercury in not only amalgams; we see it in vaccines in the form of thimerosal, which is a preservative which has never been tested, that's going into our children's bodies and because the entire food chain that you're talking about and the amount of mercury that's going into our streams not only from amalgams, but from coal-fired generators and electrical plants and so forth, we've got a serious problem.

We've gone from 1 in 10,000 children that are autistic in this country to 1 in 150. Now, something's causing that. It's not something that's just happened. They say, well, maybe it's because we haven't been keeping accurate records in the past. Well, let's say that was 1 in 5,000 before, or 1 in 2,000; now it's 1 in 150. And we have senior citizens that more and more are getting Alzheimer's disease. And the scientists that have been before our committee say that one of the contributing factors of Alzheimer's and autism is the amount of mercury that's being ingested into people's bodies, either through needles or through amalgams or other things. And I just can't understand why everybody continues to defend this substance saying, you know, it's something that's absolutely essential to be used in the art of dentistry.

I mean, I know that it is more expensive to use other substances. But if they were used in larger amounts, perhaps the cost would come down. And in any event, it seems to me that we ought to try to err on the side of safety, and we seem to be hell-bent for leather not to do that.

Are there any other questions that I need to ask this panel? Yes.

There was an article that was put out. It says, "U.S. Congressional Hearing on Dental Mercury Leaked Document Shows ADA Undercuts Pollution Exposure Reduction," say advocates. And I'd like to read you a little bit of this and then you can make a comment, Dr. Eichmiller.

It says, "As the American Dental Association prepares to testify before a U.S. congressional committee today on dental mercury, advocates released a confidential document showing the association's continuing intent to undermine efforts to reduce dental mercury pollution and human exposure from mercury fillings."

"It's like pulling teeth to get the ADA to support efforts to reduce mercury pollution and unnecessary use even though dentists are the No. 1 contributor of mercury to the Nation's wastewater and still one of the largest mercury users in the U.S. today," said Michael Bender, Director of the Mercury Policy Project.

"Meanwhile, the latest Centers of Disease Control data indicate that 8 percent of U.S. women of child-bearing age have mercury levels so high that their developing babies are at risk of neurological damage."

ADA has submitted a confidential document to EPA that, in essence, argues that reducing dental mercury pollution through installation of amalgam separators, which can capture between 95 to 99 percent of the dental mercury particles is not cost effective or necessary. In the document, ADA urges EPA to issue guidance practically devoid of amalgam separators that would recommend, "only voluntary best-management practice," unless the environmental conditions or State law mercury require mercury reductions.

Is that true?

Dr. EICHMILLER. I can speak probably to the, one of the first points that was made there.

Mr. BURTON. Well, before you go to the first point, let me go to that last point.

Did the ADA submit a confidential document to the EPA that, in essence, argues that reducing dental mercury pollution through installation of amalgam separators is not cost effective or necessary?

Dr. EICHMILLER. I'm going to defer that to Jerome here, who has been working directly with the EPA on this.

Mr. BURTON. Well, it's a simple yes or no answer. Was that sent to the EPA saying it was not cost effective?

Mr. BOWMAN. Mr. Chairman, we've made a proposal to partner with the EPA on a nationwide basis to address a series of issues relating to amalgam wastewater—amalgam discharges in wastewater, including recycling, including separators, including education.

It is the position of the ADA, and the position we have taken to EPA, that there may well be environmental conditions, local environmental conditions that warrant something over and above voluntary BMPs. But absent those environmental conditions, it is our position that voluntary best-management practices are effective and suffice.

Mr. BURTON. OK. Let me just stop you right there.

You know, if you were talking about something that was contained in a very small area, like Indianapolis, IN, for instance, where I live, or Crawfordsville, IN, it would be one thing. But this mercury gets into the water streams, the groundwater supply; it gets into the air when you burn this wastewater product, and it goes everywhere. And it gets into the fish we eat. And so, for the ADA to contact the EPA—and evidently you're admitting that happened, that you submitted a confidential document that argues that reducing dental mercury pollution through installation of amalgam separators is not cost effective or necessary—so the answer is yes, in effect, that's what you sent to the EPA, right?

Mr. BOWMAN. Mr. Chairman, if I could just point out the next clause in what you were just referring to, specific environmental conditions.

Mr. BURTON. OK. In the document, ADA urges EPA to issue guidance practically devoid of amalgam separators that would recommend only voluntary BMPs unless environmental conditions or State law requires mercury reductions.

Mr. BOWMAN. Correct.

Mr. BURTON. Yes. But the fact of the matter is, you did send a document, or documents, that said to that effect what I just read.

And so you're saying, unless the local people, like in the State of Washington, say, you've got to do this, then it's going to be on a voluntary basis? And the State of Washington said, when it was voluntary, after 6 years, 24 out of 900 dentists complied. That's a very, very small number. And since we know that 40 percent of the mercury that's going into our environment from—through the wastewater treatment plants is from dental amalgams, why in the world wouldn't you want to say to your dentists around the country, this is something you must do?

Mr. BOWMAN. Mr. Chairman, if local authorities mandate separators, the American Dental Association will do everything it can to assist our members in obtaining and installing the correct separators.

Furthermore, there are in place regulatory schemes that address surface water contaminant levels and sludge limits. If those limits or those levels are exceeded, again the American Dental Association is ready to assist our members to do what—to do their fair share to help the environment. But where there is no specific environmental problem, it is our position that voluntary methods are sufficient and work well, yes.

Mr. BURTON. You know, that—I don't want to make light of what you said, but unless there's an environmental problem—any amount of mercury in the environment's not good. Any amount of mercury in your body's not good. It's just not.

Do we have anybody here from the EPA?

Mr. KUZMACK. Yes, my name is Arnold Kuzmack.

Mr. BURTON. Did you get the document from the ADA about this? Are you familiar with that?

Mr. KUZMACK. Yes, I am familiar with the document.

Mr. BURTON. What is the EPA's response to that document?

Mr. KUZMACK. What we're doing is, we have had a meeting with ADA and then we're continuing to have additional meetings to develop areas where we can cooperate. We do continue to support local and State agencies that want to either voluntarily or on a mandatory basis require separators. We would support that, and we would not——

Mr. BURTON. On a voluntary basis?

Mr. KUZMACK. Or on a mandatory basis, depending on——

Mr. BURTON. Oh, would EPA prefer mandatory?

Mr. KUZMACK. I think as long as it works, we don't care which way they do it.

Mr. BURTON. Well, when you just heard this figure that was quoted by the gentleman from the State of Washington that—let's see, how much was it; 24 out of 900 over a 6-year period complied in a voluntary.

Does that sound to you like it's effective?

Mr. KUZMACK. In that case, obviously not. I believe there are other situations where they have been relatively effective.

Mr. BURTON. Really? Where?

Mr. KUZMACK. Duluth, MN, for example.

Mr. BURTON. How many complied on a voluntary basis?

Mr. KUZMACK. I don't have the figures in my head right now.

Mr. BURTON. Was it a high percentage?

Mr. KUZMACK. My understanding is, it was a high percentage.

Mr. BURTON. Fifty percent?

Mr. KUZMACK. I really couldn't say.

Mr. BURTON. Could you send me some statistical data on that to show that?

Mr. KUZMACK. I'll try to find something, yes.

Mr. BURTON. Would you do that?

Mr. KUZMACK. Yes, sir.

Mr. BURTON. OK.

Dr. EICHMILLER. We do have the information from the Duluth group, and it was near 100 percent compliance.

Mr. BURTON. On a voluntary basis up there?

Dr. EICHMILLER. That's correct.

Mr. BURTON. I wonder why it was only 24 out of 900 in the State of Washington.

Dr. EICHMILLER. I think that was an unfortunate situation where there was a lot of misunderstanding on both the side of the regulators and the regulated community.

We've learned an awful lot from that, and that's one of the reasons why we have made such an effort to work with the regulators since then to try to put our constituent societies in touch with them, so they can come up together with a collaborative scheme.

Mr. BURTON. OK.

Do you know who paid for the Duluth separators? Were they paid for by the individual dentists?

Mr. Berglund.

Dr. EICHMILLER. I'm not sure.

Mr. BERGLUND. Mr. Chair, I'm not sure about each and every single separator, but a good number of them were provided by the Western Lake Superior Sanitary District, the sewer board in Duluth.

Mr. BURTON. So the government up there was paying for them?

Mr. BERGLUND. Right. Yeah, a good chunk of them. The person working in Duluth acquired some grant money and funded the acquisition. Some of the separators were given to Duluth by one of the manufacturers on a trial basis and in Duluth.

Mr. BURTON. Thank you.

The gentleman from EPA, did you know they were paid for in large part by the government up there?

Mr. KUZMACK. I was not specifically aware.

I guess I'm not supporting—I'm not opposing mandatory requirements, but we are not requiring that either. If it works, it works.

Mr. BURTON. Well, the point is—and I don't know what your position is as far as authority over at the EPA is concerned, but if the ADA is coming to you with a voluntary approach and you see that in the State of Washington only a very small percentage of them complied, and then they use, as an example, another area where almost 100 percent complied, but the government was paying for the separators, you'd say, well, wait a minute. Of course, if somebody's buying me a car, I'd say, gee, that's great; I'll drive more safely.

But the fact of the matter is, we're not going to be able to pay for all the dentists in the country to have these separators. It's going to have to be mandated by somebody; otherwise, it's going to get into the wastewater treatment.

Now, let me just ask you one last question, and I'll let you gentlemen go, because I don't want to prolong this. It's getting rather late in the day.

If we didn't have mercury in our fillings, would this be a problem? Of course not. That's the answer.

If there's any question about the safety of the mercury in your mouth, why not get it out? If there's any question about the safety as far as sewage treatment plants are concerned, then why not get it out? If there's any question about the burning of it and its getting into the environment where we breathe it, then why not get it out? If there's any question about its getting into the waterways, then why not get it out?

The only question is, and it's the same thing we found with the pharmaceutical companies as far as thimerosal and the vaccines; it's money. It's money. And it's unfortunate that the safety and the health of the American people comes down to the dollar because, you know, if there's any question about it, you ought to get that substance out of there. That's the question. You ought to get it out of there.

And with that, I really, really appreciate your being here. This will not be the last hearing. We're going to have hearings around the country on this subject, and I hope that some day we'll see these things bear fruit.

We stand adjourned.

[Whereupon, at 5:36 p.m., the subcommittee was adjourned.]

[The prepared statement of Hon. Diane E. Watson follows:]

Opening Remarks of Congresswoman Diane E. Watson
Ranking Minority Member
Subcommittee Human Rights and Wellness

October 8, 2003

Thank You Mr. Chairman. The Human Rights and Wellness hearing today is very important for the American people. This hearing will provide more information about the effects of elemental mercury and its use in dental fillings. In previous hearings we have discussed different aspects about the last remaining use of mercury inside the human body, but the environmental effects of mercury are equally disturbing.

Mercury is listed as the #1 environmental poison by the World Health Organization. The Environmental Protection Agency has listed mercury as #1 of the 19 most persistent and bio-accumulative toxic metals. Last Thursday, October 2, 2003, Ballou Senior High School was shut down in South East Washington D.C. due to 250 milliliters, or approximately 450 fillings worth of mercury. I understand the public concern over the mercury spill, but we should

also be concerned with approximately ½ gram of the same

hazardous material being placed in the mouths of our children and

adults in each amalgam filling.

In a recent report entitled "Dentists the Menace", dentists were

called the biggest mercury polluters in the United States. Consider

these facts: Dentistry is one of the only unregulated major sources of

mercury discharges to the environment; Dental fillings constitute the

largest source of direct mercury pollution in wastewater; Dentistry

is the fifth largest consumer of mercury in the U.S.; and Dentists use

toxic mercury in silver fillings-which are made of 43-54% mercury.

Dentists improperly dispose of mercury dental fillings every

day. Mercury dental fillings are put in the trash that eventually will

be incinerated, releasing poisonous gasses and vapors into the air.

Properly cremated loved ones release the same mercury

contaminants into the air through mercury fillings. Dentists also discard mercury dental fillings by putting them in landfills, contaminating the soil and surrounding water sources. Mercury dental fillings pose too much risk for not only the health of dental patients but environmental and agricultural safety.

Mercury is constantly being discharged into our environment, polluting our water sources. The body tissue of fish easily absorbs mercury suspended in water. Ultimately we eat this toxic mercury. Pregnant women are constantly being warned not to eat shark, swordfish or mackerel due to their extremely high accumulation of mercury. If they are warned not to eat fish, why are they not constantly being warned to not use mercury dental fillings?

Mr. Speaker I look forward to the testimony today and I yield back my time.

○